GENETICS
FOR THE HEALTH SCIENCES

A HANDBOOK FOR CLINICAL HEALTHCARE

GENETICS

FOR THE HEALTH SCIENCES

A HANDBOOK FOR CLINICAL HEALTHCARE

HEATHER SKIRTON
Professor of Applied Health Genetics, University of Plymouth, UK

CHRISTINE PATCH
Consultant Genetic Counsellor, Clinical Genetics Department
Guy's and St Thomas' NHS Foundation Trust, London, UK

Scion

Second edition © Scion Publishing Ltd, 2009

First edition entitled *Genetics for Healthcare Professionals*, published 2002 by BIOS Scientific Publishers Ltd (ISBN 1 85996 043 X)

A CIP catalogue record for this book is available from the British Library.

ISBN 978 1 904842 70 5

Scion Publishing Ltd
Bloxham Mill, Barford Road, Bloxham, Oxfordshire OX15 4FF
www.scionpublishing.com

Important Note from the Publisher
The information contained within this book was obtained by Scion Publishing Ltd from sources believed by us to be reliable. However, while every effort has been made to ensure its accuracy, no responsibility for loss or injury whatsoever occasioned to any person acting or refraining from action as a result of information contained herein can be accepted by the authors or publishers.

The reader should remember that medicine is a constantly evolving science and while the authors and publishers have ensured that all dosages, applications and practices are based on current indications, there may be specific practices which differ between communities. You should always follow the guidelines laid down by the manufacturers of specific products and the relevant authorities in the country in which you are practising.

Typeset by Phoenix Photosetting, Chatham, Kent, UK
Printed in Great Britain by Henry Ling Limited, at the Dorset Press, Dorchester, DT1 1HD

Contents

Preface

When we wrote the first version of this book, *Genetics for Healthcare Professionals*, we were aiming to provide an accessible textbook for those healthcare practitioners who were not necessarily working in the field of genetics, but who required an understanding of genetics to perform their professional roles.

Since that time, the applications of genetics and genomics have become more widespread, with the result that more nurses, midwives and allied health professionals feel the need to have a basic knowledge of genetic science as well as the applications of current technologies in their professional setting.

We were keen to update the original book to reflect changes in knowledge and practice since 2001, but we were also aware that the readers of this book may be working in any one of a wide range of countries and disciplines. We have therefore tried to adopt an approach that makes the content applicable to practitioners wherever they are based. Because our own knowledge was developed through many years of clinical work, the emphasis is on practical issues related to the healthcare of individuals and families. Case examples are used extensively throughout the book and we have tried to address the ethical issues that arise in practice. We felt that while much of the structure of the original book has been retained, the changes have been sufficient to merit altering the title to reflect the broader focus.

We are extremely grateful to our publisher, Jonathan Ray, for his support in producing this second version of the book. We hope that readers will find this book helpful in supporting them to attain the competence required for effective healthcare.

Heather Skirton and Christine Patch

About the authors

Heather Skirton is a registered nurse and qualified midwife. She worked in pediatrics and midwifery for many years before becoming a genetic nurse. She was instrumental in introducing a registration system for genetic counsellors in the UK and is a registered genetic counsellor. Heather has over 16 years' experience in clinical genetics and she was Co-Director of the Masters course in Genetic Counselling at Cardiff University for four years. As a past President of the International Society of Nurses in Genetics and director of many European courses in genetics, she has contact with genetics health professionals worldwide. She is now Professor of Applied Health Genetics at the University of Plymouth (UK).

Christine Patch is currently Consultant Genetic Counsellor/Manager in the Clinical Genetics department in Guy's Hospital in London. She originally qualified as a nurse and started in genetics in the late 1980s. After some 15 years of experience in clinical genetics, she spent some time as a researcher before moving back into the NHS. Her research interests are in evaluating genetic technologies. She is a member and past member of various professional and advisory bodies including the UK Human Genetics Commission and the Professional and Public Policy Committee of the European Society for Human Genetics.

Notes to readers on the format of this book

- Seven families are used to illustrate a number of issues throughout the book. Where these 'core' families are discussed, the text is presented in a shaded box. Other case examples are in unshaded boxes.
- Key practice points are included in boxes in the text, to emphasize important clinical concepts.
- An extensive glossary is included at the end of the book. Where a word is encountered for the first time in the text, it is marked in bold to indicate that it is included in the glossary.
- At the end of each chapter there is a list of resources for those who wish to extend their knowledge for clinical practice.
- All websites cited in the text are posted at www.scionpublishing.com/geneticsforthehealthsciences, along with many others that may be useful to you.
- Many people have a preference for use of the terms 'patient' or 'client'. While we acknowledge that in many cases those with a genetic condition will be receiving healthcare and could be described as patients, many others are well and the use of the term patient is not appropriate. For consistency, in this book we have chosen to use the word 'client' throughout. We also feel that this is more in keeping with our own approach, which emphasizes the expertise and experience of the client as well as that of the health professional.
- There are differences in the spelling of counseling/counselling and counselor/counsellor in various countries. For consistency, we have used counselor and counseling throughout the text, except when citing documents or references where the alternative version is correct.
- The use of the possessive form of eponymous disease names (such as Huntington's disease and Down's syndrome) is now considered incorrect and we have dropped the 'apostrophe s' where relevant, hence the use of Huntington disease and Down syndrome.

Helpful websites

In the 'Further resources' section at the end of each chapter we have listed relevant websites. There is also a larger list of websites available at www.scionpublishing.com/geneticsforthehealthsciences. However, there are a number of core sites that will be generally useful, and we list them here. It is worth looking at them and saving relevant ones to your 'favourites' list.

EuroGentest project site – www.eurogentest.org/
Website for the European project on genetic testing, with a repository of relevant documents, information and downloadable patient information leaflets in many languages.

Genetic Interest Group – www.gig.org.uk/ and
Genetic Alliance – www.geneticalliance.org/
Resources on patient support groups.

Gene Tests/Gene Reviews – www.genetests.org/
Current information on genetic conditions and the tests available for those conditions.

National Coalition for Health Professional Education in Genetics
– www.nchpeg.org/
Coalition of professional and lay organizations focussed on genetics education.

National Genetics Education and Development Centre –
www.geneticseducation.nhs.uk/
Includes many resources and links for learning about and teaching genetics for healthcare practice.

Online Mendelian Inheritance in Man –
www.ncbi.nlm.nih.gov/Omim/
Authoritative information on every genetic condition.

Telling Stories: Understanding Real Life Genetics –
www.geneticseducation.nhs.uk/tellingstories/indextesting.asp
Patient stories linked to relevant educational content to enable practitioners to develop competence in genetics.

1 Setting the scene

1.1 Introduction to the book

This book has been written for all health professionals who have an interest in genetics. Since the first edition was published, there have been many changes in genetics and genomics, with increased awareness of the role that genetics plays in routine healthcare. However, education and training in genetic principles and practice has not kept pace with the demands of clinical need.

In the past, genetics was a subject confined to a number of rare conditions, and the number of families who required these explanations was relatively small. However, we now understand, through the science of genomics, that many diseases are the result of interactions between our genes and the environment in which we develop and live. In addition, it has become clearer that genes influence the ways in which we metabolize and respond to medication. A knowledge of genetics is therefore required by health professionals involved in the delivery of many aspects of healthcare.

Genetics has changed the face of medicine by introducing a 'new taxonomy of disease'[1]. Diagnosis of a range of conditions is based on genetic rather than biochemical or other forms of testing. Whilst **gene therapy** is still not in widespread clinical use, **gene** testing is now being used to identify clients at high risk of bowel[2] and breast cancer[3], so clinical screening can be targeted. Genetic testing is also used to identify specific forms of common diseases such as diabetes, so that treatment can be effectively planned[4]. The widespread use of antenatal **maternal serum screening**[5] means that every midwife needs to be aware of the use of genetic tests and the benefits and limitations of such tests. The changing health scene reflects the increasing influence of genetics, but the education of health professionals has not kept pace with these changes.

The aim of this book is to enable those working in healthcare to update their knowledge on topics related to genetics and genomics that have an impact in their daily work and apply it usefully in patient care. For this reason, the book has been written for those who work in settings where they see clients **affected** by or at risk of a genetic disease, or clients who are at low risk but will be offered screening tests for genetic conditions. That group of professionals includes those working in primary care, such as midwives and health visitors, as well as those whose role is based in specialized secondary settings such as oncology, neurology, ophthalmics, reproductive medicine, and paediatrics. The book is also appropriate for those who have an interest in genetics and wish to deepen their own knowledge. The content includes the material that is necessary for professionals to develop the basic competences in genetics that are essential for everyday practice.

The information is organized in chapters relating to particular life stages. Throughout the book, case examples will be used to demonstrate the clinical application of the topic under discussion and the seven families introduced in this first chapter will be used to explore clinical situations. An extensive glossary is included at the end of the book, with definitions of any terms that may be unfamiliar, and relevant websites are listed with other resources in the 'Further resources' section at the end of each chapter. In this chapter, some important concepts related to genetic health care will be discussed to set the scene.

1.2 Defining genetic counseling

A current definition of genetic counseling was produced in 2006 by a Task Force appointed by the US-based National Society of Genetic Counselors (NSGC)[6]. The definition states that:

> "Genetic counseling is the process of helping people understand and adapt to the medical, psychological and familial implications of genetic contributions to disease. This process integrates the following: Interpretation of family and medical histories to assess the chance of disease occurrence or recurrence. Education about inheritance, testing, management, prevention, resources and research. Counseling to promote informed choices and adaptation to the risk or condition."

This is a more succinct definition than that produced by the American Society for Human Genetics in 1975[7], but includes the same principles. Although over 30 years has passed since that was first written, it still accurately reflects the extent of services provided under the title 'genetic counseling'.

1.3 Genetic services

Genetic services are provided in many countries by a variety of health professionals. One model of care is based on the provision of clinical genetic services by a multi-disciplinary team that includes medical geneticists and genetic nurses and/or **genetic counselors**. Most families are referred to the genetic service by either the family doctor or a specialist (e.g. pediatrician, neurologist or obstetrician) caring for the affected or at-risk person, although in some countries families can self-refer.

The types of families referred for genetic services fall into four main groups.

1.	Families who are concerned about a known or suspected genetic condition such as cystic fibrosis, Huntington disease or muscular dystrophy.

2.	Where there is concern about a child in the family who has learning **delay** and/or **dysmorphic features.**

3.	After the diagnosis of fetal abnormality or fetal loss during a pregnancy, or in the neonatal period, or recurrent **spontaneous abortion.**

4.	Families where there is a strong history of cancer.

The following referrals are typical of those received in any genetics department, and these families will be used throughout the book to illustrate the principles discussed. Other family examples will be given where relevant.

Harding Family

Dear Doctor

Re: Sarah Harding, age 28 years

I would be grateful if you could see Sarah and offer her some advice regarding her family history of Huntington disease. Sadly, Sarah's mother suffers from this condition and Sarah is now wondering whether she could be tested, especially as she is expecting her first baby. We would welcome your expert advice.

Yours,

Community Midwife

Collins Family

Dear Doctor

Re: Carol Collins, age 33 years
     Adam Collins, age 11 years

Carol has been in the surgery today with her son Adam aged 11. In the course of the consultation for another reason she mentioned that she'd been told that Adam would need a bowel check from about now. Carol herself had a total colectomy some years ago and still has regular check-ups at the hospital.

She tells me that this is a genetic condition and when she had her operation she was told the children should be screened when they reached the age of 10.

I would be grateful if you would see and advise.

GP

Singh Family

Telephone referral received from neonatal pediatrician, notes taken by the secretary are:

Baby Singh
  Born today, small for dates
  Cleft palate
  Possible cardiac defect
  Low serum calcium levels
  Please give an opinion

Spencer Family

Dear Doctor

Re: Luke Spencer, age 4 years

I have been seeing this little boy because of his language delay. I recently checked his chromosomes and the result has shown that he has the fragile X syndrome. His mother would like to discuss this.

Community Pediatrician

Chester Family

Dear Genetic Counselor

Could you please see Colin Chester and his wife Julie. Their second child, Samuel, is 3 months old and has been diagnosed with cystic fibrosis through the newborn screening program. Samuel is doing well and is under the care of the CF Specialist team. Colin and Julie are thinking about their next pregnancy and would like to discuss risks and options with you.

Sincerely,

Family Doctor

Levy Family

Dear Surgeon

Mrs Levy has come to me today worried about a lump in her breast. Could you arrange the appropriate investigations?

Mrs Levy has a family history of breast cancer so I have copied this letter to the genetics team to ask them to assess her risk.

Yours sincerely,

Family Doctor

Campbell Family

Dear Doctor

Mr David Campbell came to see me today with his partner. He is now aged 31 years and considering having children. He is extremely concerned because his sister and an uncle have both been diagnosed with schizophrenia, the uncle many years ago.

His experience with his sister has made him reluctant to have a family if the chances of him developing it or his children inheriting it are high. He recently read about a genetic test and would like to have it. Could you see him to discuss?

Yours truly,

Practice Nurse

Although the service for individual families varies according to need and the condition concerned, in general the following aspects of care will be offered by the genetic service.

Diagnosis. Whilst this seems an obvious starting point, in many situations the correct diagnosis of an affected member may not be known because of limited medical knowledge at the time the person became symptomatic, or their reluctance to pursue the diagnosis. In order to treat an affected person, the exact mode of inheritance may not be relevant, but it is a critical piece of information if you are to advise family members about the risk to themselves or their offspring. Let's think about Melanie, a young woman who presents asking about the risk of muscular dystrophy. Her brother aged 20 years is affected, and she is worried about her future children. She says her brother has muscular dystrophy, but this could be one of many types, with different patterns of inheritance, including the following.

i.   Duchenne muscular dystrophy, an **X-linked** condition. Women can be **carriers**, and if she were a carrier then each male child of hers would have a 50% risk of having the condition.

ii. Myotonic dystrophy, a **dominant** condition. She could have very mild signs and if she were affected, then both male and female children would have a 50% risk of inheriting muscular dystrophy. Her children might be at risk of a very severe congenital type.

iii. Emery–Dreifuss muscular dystrophy. This is an **autosomal recessive** condition and, even if she were affected, her children would be at low risk because the chances that her partner also carried the condition would be very low.

Finding the correct genetic basis of the muscular dystrophy is necessary to give Melanie the correct information about the risks to her future children and the potential for prenatal testing. Similarly, a family history of cancer must be confirmed to enable correct risk estimates and accurate advice about screening to be given. This is covered in detail in *Chapter 10*.

Information giving. This includes:
- mode of inheritance
- natural history of the condition
- signs and symptoms
- prognosis.

Evaluation of risk and discussion and explanation of that risk to each interested family member.

Presentation of appropriate options, including:
- preventive / lifestyle measures, such as the use of folic acid pre-conceptually to reduce risk of **neural tube defects**
- testing, including diagnostic, pre-symptomatic, predictive and prenatal
- clinical surveillance, such as mammography, renal scans or monitoring of blood pressure

Ongoing contact and support. Genetic counseling does not generally include treatment or management of the genetic condition, which is usually organized by the relevant speciality service. However, some genetic conditions are extremely rare and many other health professionals will have limited experience of the condition. These conditions may also be complex, involving multiple body systems (e.g. von Hippel Lindau syndrome). In these cases, affected individuals may attend a specific genetic clinic to be seen by a genetic specialist who has expertise in management of that condition. Joint clinics involving a geneticist and other relevant specialists are increasingly common and enable clients to discuss a range of issues at the same appointment.

1.4 Types of genetic testing

1.4.1 *What is a genetic test?*

There has been much discussion about the definition of a genetic test, particularly in the context of the type of counseling and information that should accompany a test. There is one opinion that states that any test involving **DNA** or **chromosome** studies may be considered a genetic test, although some such tests do not actually provide information about the person's genetic identity. A good example is the use of chromosome studies in the diagnosis of leukemia, where the Philadelphia chromosome is an indicator of the presence of the disease rather than an inherited characteristic. However, others believe that a genetic test should be defined as one that has implications for more than one person. A 'routine' test, such as a full blood count or renal scan, may reveal information that has relevance for both the individual and other members of the family if it shows a diagnosis of sickle cell anemia or polycystic kidneys. A helpful working definition of a genetic test is therefore any test, the result of which would prompt the health professional concerned to alert other family members of potential risk. In reality, the health professional would normally ask the original patient to inform the family, rather than contacting the family personally, but it is the principle of broader contact that is important rather than the practicalities.

1.4.2 Diagnostic test

Diagnostic genetic tests are those performed where there is already a clinical suspicion of disease, and the test is performed to confirm or identify the disease.

1.4.3 Predictive / pre-symptomatic test

In the literature, there is some discussion about the use of the terms predictive and pre-symptomatic and they are sometimes used inter-changeably. Both refer to a situation where a person has not yet developed any symptoms or signs of the condition. In this book, we will use the definitions used by the European-wide project to standardize genetic testing[8], which states that the term 'pre-symptomatic test' refers to those tests performed where the onset of the disease is considered inevitable. The term 'predictive test' is now used to describe a test that indicates the presence of a disease gene, but where the onset of signs and symptoms is not certain.

Because these conditions are usually those that occur in adulthood, predictive and pre-symptomatic tests are rarely carried out on minors. Freedom to choose whether to be tested, and psychological preparation for the result, are considered important (see *Chapter 9*).

1.4.4 Prenatal test

This applies to any genetic test performed to provide information about the status of the fetus, and includes results of ultrasound **scanning**, chromosome studies performed with material obtained during **amniocentesis** or **chorionic villus biopsy,** or fetal blood sampling (see *Chapter 6*).

Genetic testing differs from **genetic screening**, which is a term sometimes used for the testing of a population in order to detect those at high risk. Genetic tests are performed for an individual at significant risk because of family history or because they are symptomatic. For example, testing the fetus of a woman who is a known carrier of Duchenne muscular dystrophy. Measuring serum creatine kinase levels of all newborn boys to detect raised levels (that may indicate the boy has a form of muscular dystrophy) is an example of population screening for a genetic condition.

1.5 Ethical practice

The ethical principles underlying 'virtue' ethics have long been the mainstay of medical ethics and these underpin the work of the genetic counselor. The main principles are:

- beneficence (the duty to do good)
- non-maleficence (the duty to prevent harm)
- justice (equity of care)
- autonomy (the belief that a person is able to act in their own best interests)

However, when working with a number of individuals within a family, these principles may not provide straightforward guidelines or solutions. These challenges have been recognized in several key initiatives in both Europe and the US. A document entitled *Consent and Confidentiality* was produced by the UK Joint Committee on Medical Genetics[9] to guide practitioners through the legal and ethical requirements of genetic testing. This document was written to ensure that practitioners were clear about the legal framework surrounding consent, the sharing of genetic information and genetic testing.

In the US, the work of health professionals is legally controlled by the Health Insurance Portability and Accountability Act (HIPAA)[10], which was enacted by Congress in 1996. This Act governs the use of medical information in records, or obtained through conversations, and prohibits the sharing and/or use of medical information without consent except in special circumstances described by the Act (these include to avoid or reduce the chance of epidemics). In general, an individual's medical information cannot be shared with relatives unless it is essential for the care of that individual. This precludes sharing information because of the potential impact on the relative's own health.

In practical terms, these difficult situations are not usually resolved quickly. The genetics team will spend time with the family discussing the options for action, and potential outcomes. For example, the counselor might ask Lindsay how he might feel if his mother became depressed after hearing the result, whilst Joan might be asked to consider how she might feel if Lindsay and his

---

ETHICAL DILEMMA 1   JOAN

Joan is 45 years old and has a 50% chance of inheriting Huntington disease (HD) from her mother. Her son Lindsay wants to be tested for the gene **mutation** that causes HD. He is married and wants to know his own status before deciding to have a family.

A positive result for Lindsay would inform Joan that she has also inherited the mutation. Joan dreads having HD and feels she would not cope if she knew that was awaiting her.

Benefiting Lindsay could result in harm to Joan.

ETHICAL DILEMMA 2 CHLOE

Chloe is a 26 year old whose father has the X-linked condition, Becker muscular dystrophy. Chloe has studied genetics and realizes that all daughters of a man with an X-linked condition will be obligate carriers.

Chloe is pregnant and requests prenatal diagnosis so that she can avoid having a son with the condition. Her mother telephones the genetic counselor to say that Chloe was born after donor insemination, but she is not aware of this and her father does not want her to know as he feels it will change their close relationship.

Unless Chloe is made aware that it is unlikely she is a carrier, she may undergo an unnecessary invasive diagnostic procedure that puts the pregnancy at risk.

ETHICAL DILEMMA 3 ROY

Roy is found to have a balanced chromosome **translocation** after his wife has three spontaneous abortions. If one parent carries a translocation, there is an increased risk in every pregnancy of either having a child with physical and mental disabilities or spontaneous abortion.

Roy has a sister, who may also carry the translocation. He refuses to tell her of his carrier status and alert her to the potential risks to her own future children.

Respecting Roy's autonomy by maintaining his confidentiality may conflict with the rights of his sister to prevent the birth of a child with a serious disability.

wife decided they could not risk starting a family without having a test. Often over a period of time the family will resolve the conflict by finding a compromise. When Lindsay realized how his mother felt, he agreed to wait until she was 50 before being tested. As Joan's mother was affected by the age of 40 years, if Joan had inherited HD she was likely to be symptomatic by that time. Joan agreed to this plan, as she did not wish to deny Lindsay the chance to find out and felt she had time to prepare for knowing her status.

In Chloe's case, the genetic counselor was given the information about Chloe's paternity but it was confidential. She discussed the potential implications with Chloe's mother, who agreed that the information could be shared with other professionals. At the multi-disciplinary team meeting it was discussed and a decision was made to test Chloe to see if she was a carrier. Chloe was found not to be a carrier and was told prenatal diagnosis was not indicated. Chloe and her mother talked about this subsequently. Chloe was very concerned to protect her father from any hurt and they decided that they would not tell her father that she knew of her paternity.

If the family is unable to negotiate a solution, then the genetics team will discuss a course of action that causes least harm, usually seeking opinions from other experienced team members and colleagues in other regions or specialities. The opinion of a medical ethicist or lawyer might be sought, as the legal situation varies according to the country of practice. In Roy's case, he was unwilling to change his position and the law prevented the genetics team from taking any direct action to alert his sister. However, when she became pregnant she mentioned to her midwife that her sister-in-law had lost three pregnancies. The midwife contacted the genetic counselor, who advised a chromosome analysis for the sister, based on that family history and without disclosing that she knew Roy. The sister had a normal **karyotype** and no further action was needed.

It is important to work in a way that is in the best interests of the client and minimizes harm, but the professional's responsibility does not extend to resolving conflict or disputes within a family. The professional also needs to respect the way in which the family deals with the situation subsequently, even where this might create discomfort.

1.6 Genetic testing of children

Genetic testing of children is another potentially controversial area of practice. Children are generally not tested unless the result will in some way benefit the health of the child before they reach adulthood, and so it may be considered to be in the child's 'best interests'. If the test result will only be of significance in adulthood, then the test is usually deferred until the child is able to give informed consent. Informed consent implies that the person consenting has understood the reason for the test and the implications of the result.

In some cases, genetic testing in childhood will be of benefit to the child. There are often benefits from making a diagnosis in a child with a genetic **syndrome**, as there may be problems associated with the syndrome that would warrant extra surveillance or treatment.

CASE EXAMPLE   SAMANTHA

A child called Samantha was referred to the genetic service because of her learning problems at school. She was falling behind her classmates in Year Two. A chromosome study showed she had a **microdeletion** of chromosome 22, which can cause learning difficulties, speech delay and heart abnormalities. Samantha had an echocardiogram that showed she had a mild heart defect, and she was treated by the pediatric cardiologist. She was also referred for speech therapy, and because of her diagnosis was granted additional help at school.

In some cases, the child may be at risk of a condition for which invasive screening is recommended. Genetic testing for the child may clarify the need for such screening.

Collins Family

*Robert and Gemma are the two children of Michael, the brother of Carol Collins, who has Familial Adenomatous Polyposis (FAP). This is a condition in which multiple **polyps** grow in the colon, predisposing the affected person to colorectal cancer. Screening by **colonoscopy** is usually arranged for such children annually from the age of 12 years. A genetic test that clarifies whether the children have inherited the gene mutation from their father would either confirm the need for invasive screening, or remove the necessity for the screening. In this case, genetic testing is clearly in the best interests of the children. However, the test would usually be undertaken as late as possible before screening starts, to give the children the opportunity to discuss it fully and give their consent. In this family, Gemma was tested at 11 years and was found to have the mutation. She had screening annually and had a colectomy at 17 years of age. Robert was tested the following year, when he was 10 years, at his request. He had not inherited the mutation and screening was not necessary for him.*

When making a decision about what is in the 'best interests' of the child, psychological health must also be considered. The child or young person may actually experience more harm through living with uncertainty. In certain cases, a young person who has known of his/her genetic risk for many years will request a carrier test before they are 18 years of age. Provided the request comes from the young person, and they are able to give informed consent, the request for testing will probably be seriously considered. Guidelines on the testing of children have been written by the Clinical Genetics Society (UK) and copies are available from them (www.clingensoc.org).

1.7 Genetics and insurance

There has been considerable debate in the literature and media about the potential for discrimination, in both employment and insurance, if predictive genetic testing is carried out. The concern is that if an individual has a genetic test that shows an increased risk of specific illnesses developing, then that individual may be unable to purchase insurance. However, it should be borne in mind that if an individual discloses a family history of a genetic condition, this in itself will have an impact on obtaining insurance and the premiums charged; it is not only genetic testing that affects the situation, but family history. Since most insurance application forms include questions on family history, it is not possible to avoid providing this information, and to knowingly withhold it may make the insurance invalid.

It should be remembered that the potential impact of genetic discrimination will be very different according to public policy in individual countries. For example, in the USA where much of the concern is expressed, many of the population depend on private insurance for their healthcare provision and, consequently, an alteration in risk will have implications for their insurability. In 2008, a law entitled the Genetic Information Nondiscrimination Act[11] was passed by the US Senate to protect those at risk of discrimination due to their genetic status. The law will: '(a) prohibit the use of genetic information to deny employment or insurance coverage; (b) ensure that genetic test results are kept private; and (c) prevent an insurer from basing eligibility or premiums on genetic information'.

In the UK, where healthcare is universally funded through taxation (at the present time) and free at the point of service, the issues of genetic testing in relation to healthcare provision are different. This may become more relevant if genetic testing for predisposition to elderly onset diseases such as dementia becomes possible, since funding for nursing home care for the elderly is constantly under review. Discussions in the UK between the government, the insurance industry, the **clinical genetics** community, consumers, and other stakeholders, have led to an extension of an original moratorium on the use of genetic tests in assessing applications for life insurance, critical illness insurance, long term care and income protection policies, up to specific financial limits. In addition, an advisory body, the Genetics and Insurance Committee, assesses the actuarial validity of any proposed genetic test, and advises on its potential usefulness. It is essential that dialogue continues between the parties involved in order to ensure that both the potential and limitations of genetic advances are fully discussed.

1.8 Impact of the genetic condition on the family

It is extremely difficult to generalize about the impact of a genetic condition on the family, because the conditions, circumstances and families differ so greatly. Perhaps the best way to approach each family is to bear in mind that one cannot predict the impact. What may be devastating for one family may be seen positively by another.

CASE EXAMPLE   JOANNE

Joanne is a genetic counselor. One day she was asked to see two different couples, both of whom had recently terminated a pregnancy.

The first couple she saw were devastated, it had been their first pregnancy and they 'had not dreamt anything could go wrong'. When the baby was diagnosed with severe **spina bifida** and **hydrocephalus** at 19 weeks gestation, they had decided to terminate the pregnancy but felt guilty, as though they had abandoned her. Joanne spent an hour with them, although little information was discussed at the time because they were so distressed. She saw this couple on three further occasions.

She went on to visit another couple who had also terminated a recent pregnancy, after a scan showed a serious heart defect. This couple were farmers who felt that an abnormal baby had a poor chance of survival, and that termination of pregnancy had spared their child additional suffering. They were already planning another pregnancy and wanted to ensure the fetus was scanned at an early stage.

For most families, however, the diagnosis of a genetic condition is accompanied by a feeling of loss. This may be related to:

- loss of a family member due to death
- loss of health
- impairment or disability
- loss of a normal future or the expectation of a normal future
- loss of independence
- loss of security

Because of the familial nature of genetic conditions, these losses often extend to the wider family, and family support systems often become stretched. Many family members report that they feel guilty, this might be because they have 'passed it on', however unknowingly, or even because they have escaped the disease while other relatives have not. Guilt remains a part of many parents' lives, and the loss of the freedom to have a family without undue worry is an aspect that features strongly in some family stories.

In any experience of loss, mourning has a part in helping the family adjust to the loss and resume life within their altered circumstances. The pace at which family members achieve this will often differ, and this may cause additional family tensions. In our experience, it is often helpful to confirm that a loss has occurred and that feelings of grief are natural. There is now much work on the power of 'telling your story'; indeed much of the therapeutic value of counseling is ascribed to providing an opportunity to discuss an issue with another person who is empathetic but not directly affected by the situation. For professionals working with those at risk of a genetic condition, allowing time to listen to the story can be genuinely beneficial to the family.

1.9 Non-directiveness in genetic health care

The aim of genetic counseling is broadly to enable individuals and families at genetic risk to live as normal a life as possible. However, the focus is very much on the family's wishes. The onus is therefore upon the genetic counselor to present the available options in a non-judgemental way and to facilitate the client to make the best choice for themselves, in their unique circumstances. Much has been written about the need for **non-directiveness** in genetic counseling[12] and this may be, at least in part, a reaction to the **eugenic** approaches adopted in some countries during certain periods of history[13].

Non-directiveness by the counselor is not synonymous with remaining 'uninvolved' in the client's process of decision-making. Ideally, the counselor is skilled enough to enable the client to explore the options and support them in their choice, whilst remaining non-judgemental. It is recognized that this is a challenging task, particularly if the personal values and beliefs of the counselor conflict with those of the client. For this reason, training in counseling skills that includes work on developing personal awareness is a necessary part of the preparation and ongoing education of genetic counselors. Counseling and clinical supervision are also ongoing requirements for work in this field and these are discussed in depth in *Chapter 3*.

1.10 Disability and choice

Increasingly there are ethical debates about the rights of disabled individuals and the option of choice for parents. One perspective promoted by some groups is focussed on a social construct of disability; in other words, individuals are *disabled* because of the way in which society accommodates them, or not. This view emphasizes the individuality of all members of the community, but claims that when facilities and opportunities are based on the 'able', others are disabled by the lack of consideration of their needs. There is a body of opinion that states that offering parents reproductive choices, which include termination of affected pregnancies, reduces acceptability of those that might be perceived to be disabled, and results in a decrease in facilities for those people. This is an issue on which health professionals may have a personal opinion, but the role they undertake with families should facilitate the family's choice, within the legal framework for practice. They may feel there is a conflict between supporting parental choice and affording respect and dignity to individuals who are affected by a genetic condition. Others argue that genetic testing and counseling should be available to all, including individuals with a disability[14]. Clinical and counseling supervision is essential to support practice where there is a potential for conflict and ambiguity. See *Further resources* for an article on this issue.

1.11 Conclusion

In this initial chapter, we have introduced some of the relevant concepts for health professionals who provide care for any individual or family with concerns about a genetic condition. In the following chapters, we will focus on families at different times in the life cycle, and highlight the genetic issues that are relevant for each.

Test yourself

Q1. Describe five main components of a genetic counseling interaction?

Q2. What is the difference between a diagnostic and pre-symptomatic test? How might the client's reaction to a positive result vary, depending on whether the test was diagnostic or pre-symptomatic?

Q3. Look at the referral letter for the Spencer family. What types of losses might the family be experiencing prior to a genetic appointment?

Further resources

www.bshg.org.uk/documents/official_docs/Consent_and_confid_corrected _21%5B1%5D.8.06.pdf – Consent and confidentiality in genetic practice. *Comprehensive guidance on consent and disclosure issues.*

www.genome.gov/10002077 – Genetic Information Nondiscrimination Act. *US nondiscrimination law.*

www.hhs.gov/ocr/hipaa/ – Health Insurance Portability and Accountability Act (HIPAA). *US Act referring to discrimination in health provision.*

www.ukwatch.net/article/disability_rights – 'Disability Rights' by Tom Shakespeare.

Miller SM, McDaniel SH, Rolland JS, Feetham SL. (2006) *Individuals, Families and the New Era of Genetics. Biopsychosocial perspectives.* New York: WW Norton & Co, Inc. *In depth discussion of many relevant issues in genetic healthcare.*

2 The family history

2.1 Introduction

Although there are a great number of genetic tests conducted in a laboratory, the single most important tool and test in clinical genetics is the family history. Taking an accurate family history gives the genetic counselor a wealth of information about the likelihood of a genetic condition in the family, the probable inheritance pattern, and **recurrence risks** for family members. It also has an important function in providing context for any laboratory test results, so that they can be correctly interpreted.

The ability to take a family history will be an essential skill for most health professionals reading this book! Following the guidelines given here, you should be able to attain a reasonable level of competence, but practice will help you develop more effective ways of obtaining the information needed from the client. The person seeking the genetic information is referred to as called the **consultand**. The affected person (who may also be the person seeking genetic information) is called the **proband**.

It is important to remember the ethical aspects of taking the family tree. Some of the information may be highly confidential and should not be shared with other family members unless consent is expressly given.

In the US, family history has been given a high profile by an initiative titled the 'U.S. Surgeon General's Family History Initiative'. The website supporting this development (www.hhs.gov/familyhistory/) enables any individual to complete the details on his or her family and generate a family tree, which can be used for discussion with the family or health professionals.

It is important to use a set of symbols that will be recognized by other health professionals and enable them to correctly interpret the information. A list of recognized symbols is shown in *Figure 2.1*. These are consistent with those recommended by the (UK) National Genetics Education and Development Centre and those used by the US Surgeon General's Family History Initiative.

2.2 Guidelines for drawing the family tree

Explain why you are drawing the family tree and how it will be used. Enable the client to see what you are drawing.

1. Start with the client and his/her immediate family. These will be the most familiar to him or her and the most relevant to the client's own health or risk assessment.

2. Build the tree in a structured way, asking first about one side of the family, then moving to the other side.

3. Remember to ask about pregnancy losses; you can do this by asking 'Did you lose any babies?'.

4. Clients may not remember to tell you about relatives who have died. One way to put this is 'and how many brothers and sisters *did* your mother have?', rather than 'how many brothers and sisters *does* your mother have?'.

Pedigree symbols

There is a generally accepted set of symbols that are used to convey information about the family structure via a pedigree. The word pedigree derives from the French for foot of a crane, as the original pedigrees resembled the structure of a bird's foot.

Male   Female

A filled symbol indicates that the person was or is affected by the condition

Affected male   Affected female

A diagonal line through the symbol indicates that the person is deceased

Partners are joined by an unbroken line

If the relationship has ended this is indicated by a slanted line

Pregnancy is shown as

Male baby   Female baby   Unknown baby

Figure 2.1. Pedigree symbols.

5. Clients may include information about relatives who are not related biologically. It is important to acknowledge the social structure of the family as well as the genetic structure, for this reason we include those relatives, making a note on the **pedigree** about their relationship to the client.

6. A note 'adopted' on the pedigree does not make it clear to someone else whether the relative has been adopted into the family or was given up for adoption, so ensure this is recorded.

7. Ask about **consanguinity** in the family, as this may have some bearing on recessively inherited conditions. Some clients may be sensitive to this question, but some ways of phrasing it gently are 'Do you have any grandparents in common?' or 'Were you related before marriage?".

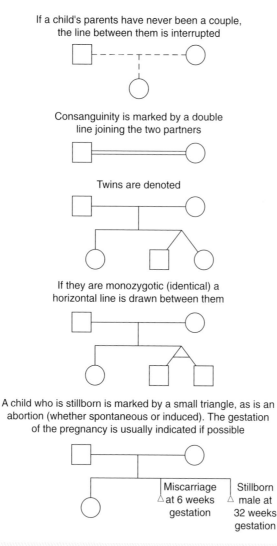

Figure 2.1. Pedigree symbols (continued).

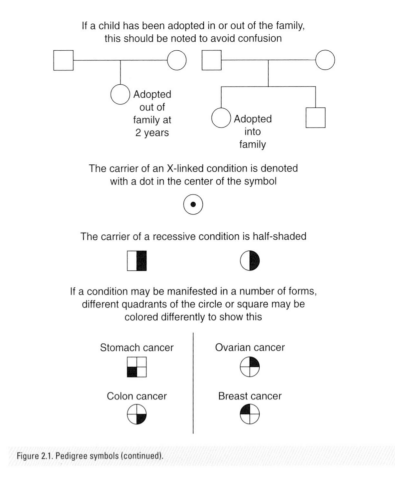

Figure 2.1. Pedigree symbols (continued).

8. A client may offer very sensitive information about previous pregnancies or paternity issues. Use your discretion about whether these are relevant for documentation purposes. Remember that you may be using the pedigree when counseling the family in future, and need some way of reminding yourself about these issues.

9. When counseling different branches of the same family, it is helpful to draw a new tree, to ascertain the information that is known by those family members. It is not uncommon to have completely different levels of information held by different family members. Discussion can then be restricted to the information held by that particular branch, without breaching confidentiality of other members of the family.

10. When you have finished drawing the tree, always ask, 'Is there anything you think I should know that we haven't mentioned?'.

More information and hints on drawing the pedigree are available on the National Genetics Education and Development Centre (NGEDC) website listed in the *Further resources*.

2.3 Drawing the tree – a practical example using the Singh family

Rajesh and Maya Singh are seen by the genetic counselor in the neonatal unit when their son is a week old. Baby Jahan had previously been seen for an initial opinion by the medical geneticist, but the parents were not present at the time. The counselor (C) has made an appointment to meet with them, to take a family history and give them information about the genetic referral. Here is a transcript of that session, following the introductions....

C: Would it be okay if we started by drawing your family tree?

Maya: We'll try, although my family is here, most of Rajesh's family are living in India or Canada now ... so we don't see them much.

C: That's fine, let's just make a start and see how we get on, most people have some gaps in their knowledge about the family ... even when they live close by ... let's start with you and Rajesh, Maya, what's your date of birth?

Maya: Mine is 10 March, 1979

C: And was Singh your name before you were married?

Maya: Yes it was, but it is a very common name in our community.

C: So your birth name was Singh as well? Is that right?

Maya: Yes, that's right. No need to change the credit card when we got married!

C: Right, that's handy ... have you ever had any serious illnesses yourself Maya?

Maya: No, my Mum told me that when I was born I had clicky hips ... she had to use special nappies on me for a while I think, apart from that, nothing really except the usual colds, flu and that

C: Okay, Rajesh, what is your date of birth?

Rajesh: 1 June, 1980

C: And have you had any serious health problems?

Rajesh: Well, how serious do you mean?

C: Have you ever needed to see a specialist or go to hospital?

Rajesh: When I was small I used to go to see a lady who was a speech therapist for a while

C: Do you know why that was? Why you saw the speech therapist?

Rajesh: Not really, it was after I started school, the teacher told Mum she thought it would help me, so I went for a few years, every so often, can't remember much about it, I was pretty young ...

C: And do you remember seeing a doctor, or a specialist?

Rajesh: No, don't think so, it was just this lady who used to come to the school

C: Okay, anything else, any serious illnesses, Rajesh?

Rajesh: No, I'm pretty fit really ...

C: Can I just ask if either of you had any problems with your learning, like did you have any special help at school?

Rajesh: Maya certainly didn't! She has a degree in history! I struggled at school, hated it, left as soon as I could but I've done okay, got an apprenticeship and now work for myself ... we do okay

C: And your baby boy was born a week ago, do you have any other children?

Maya: No, he's our first, but I did lose one before him ...

C: You lost one? How far pregnant were you?

Rajesh: Maya had a miscarriage at 15 weeks, we were really upset, so were our parents ... so he is very precious

C: He's a much wanted baby

Maya: Yes, of course all babies should be, but we feel he's very special … and now … not a good start for him …

Maya starts to cry and Rajesh puts his arm around her … the counselor waits and then they talk for a while about how worried Rajesh and Maya have been over the past week. When Maya is ready, they go on …

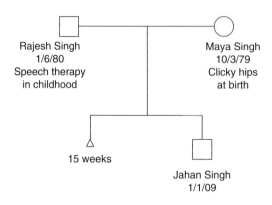

C: Now Rajesh, can I ask you about your side of the family, do you have any brothers or sisters?

Rajesh: Yes, I have one sister, ten years older than me. She is in Canada, she has 3 daughters.

C: Has your sister had any health problems herself?

Rajesh: Not really, she had problems … what was it Maya?

Maya: She had a smear test that was a bit abnormal but they did laser and she's okay now.

C: A cervical smear was that?

Maya: Yes, but that was two years ago and she's okay now …

C: And the ages of her girls?

Maya: 10, 8 and 5, they're all fine. The little one is quite a handful though, she is always in trouble! She is really naughty …

Rajesh: She's the youngest and they spoil her …

C: Is she at school yet?

Rajesh: Yes, but she's a bit slow I think, just like me!

C: And did your mother lose any children Rajesh?

Rajesh: Not that I know of … but she's very private, she wouldn't talk to me about things like that

C: What is your mother's name and date of birth?

Rajesh: Aditi Singh, 27 May, 1955

C: Is your mother in good health?

Rajesh: Yes, she has a bit of blood pressure, but nothing serious

C: And your father?

Rajesh: He died two years ago, from a heart attack, it was very sudden, I had to rush out to India to be with my mother … she has coped better than I thought though, we ask her to come here but she'd rather stay with her friends … now she has a grandson, that might make a difference …

C: Sounds like your family have had a very tough time over the past few years …
had your father had any other illnesses?

Rajesh: No, the heart attack came out of the blue

C: And his name and date of birth?

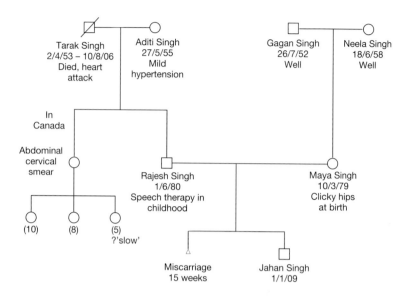

In this way, the family tree is built up, gradually moving further back in the family, at least as far back as the client's grandparents if possible. The counselor asks about Maya's family and learns she is an only child and her parents are both well, but live in another city.

In the course of taking the family history, the genetic counselor also acquires a lot of information about the nature of relationships in the family (such as who talks to whom) and the social issues that have had an impact on the family. For example, in Maya and Rajesh's family, the counselor has learnt that the couple have limited family support nearby, that there has been a major bereavement in the past two years with the sudden death of Rajesh's father, and that the couple had lost one previous pregnancy. This enhances individualized care, because the counselor is able to take family issues into account when discussing options and potential actions.

2.4 Dealing with unexpected information when taking the family tree

When taking a family tree because of the family's concern about one genetic condition, it is not uncommon to be given information of significance about another unrelated condition. For example, when seeing a family at risk of retinitis pigmentosa, an ophthalmic condition, they may talk about a history of cancer in several relatives. It is often difficult to know how to deal with this new information, as raising anxiety with no real benefit might cause harm. However, the following questions might help to clarify any action you should take.

- Is the family concerned about the condition?
- Is the family asking questions about the condition?
- Is there likely to be any significant risk to family members?
- Are the risks avoidable?
- Is there any treatment or screening available from which the family could benefit?

If the answer is yes to any of these questions, then undoubtedly the issue should be discussed with the family. If you are a professional specializing in a particular group of conditions (e.g. cancer or cardiac conditions) and you are taking a family history, it is essential that you seek advice about other potential genetic conditions before giving information to the family about the potential implications of the family history. Discussion with colleagues is necessary in these situations to clarify the best course of action.

CASE EXAMPLE   JULIA

Julia is an advanced practice nurse in an ophthalmic clinic. She takes a family history from a young couple whose child has been born with ocular albinism. The father, who is over 6 feet tall, mentions that his sister and father both had dislocated lenses. Julia is aware that dislocated lenses and tall stature are possible signs of Marfan syndrome. The family seem unaware of this. She discusses it with her colleagues and they decide that since Marfan syndrome can cause sudden early death, and screening tests and preventive surgery are available, she should discuss referring the father to a cardiologist for an assessment. When she does this, the father tells her that he has been worried about Marfan syndrome since reading about it in a newspaper article and is relieved to have an opportunity to be assessed.

2.5 Inheritance patterns

Frequently, the pattern of inheritance of a genetic condition in the family can be identified by looking at the family tree, as each of the patterns have significant characteristics.

2.5.1 Dominant conditions

If a condition is autosomal dominant, a person who inherits only one faulty copy of the particular gene involved will usually develop the condition. One normal copy of the gene is not sufficient to ensure normal cell function. Each child of an affected person has a 50% chance of inheriting the faulty gene from their affected parent. Some examples of dominant conditions are: Huntington disease, familial adenomatous polyposis (FAP), neurofibromatosis, tuberous sclerosis, adult polycystic kidney disease, and Marfan syndrome.

Features of a dominant inheritance pattern (see *Figure 2.2*):
- usually individuals in more than one successive generation are affected
- people of both sexes are affected
- male-to-male transmission can occur

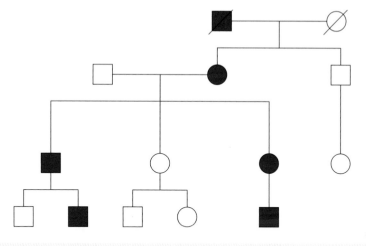

Figure 2.2. Typical dominant inheritance pattern pedigree.

2.5.2 *Recessive conditions*

A person will be affected by a recessive condition if they inherit two faulty copies of the same gene, one from each parent. If both parents are carriers, they will each have one faulty and one normal copy of the gene. Carriers are usually healthy, because having one normal copy is enough to ensure adequate cell function. Each child of two carrier parents has a 25% chance of being affected with the condition, and a 50% chance of being a carrier. Recessive conditions include cystic fibrosis, thalassemia, sickle cell disease, phenylketonuria, galactosemia, and hemochromatosis.

Features of a recessive inheritance pattern (see *Figure 2.3*):
- usually only individuals in one generation (and from one set of parents) are affected
- people of both sexes can be affected
- affected offspring usually have two unaffected parents

2.5.3 *X-linked conditions*

Conditions that are known as X-linked are caused by faulty genes on the X chromosome. Females have two X chromosomes, while males have only one. To ensure that the balance of genetic activity is the same in the cells of males and females, one X chromosome is 'turned off' in each cell in the female. This is called X-inactivation. The X chromosome that is inactive is normally randomly selected early in embryonic life, but this random inactivation can be altered in some X-linked conditions, when 'skewed inactivation' is said to occur.

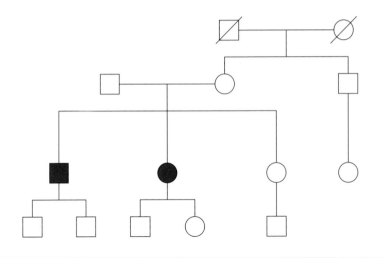

Figure 2.3. Typical recessive inheritance pattern pedigree.

Most X-linked conditions are X-linked recessive, which means that a woman will usually not develop the condition, as she will have both a normal and a faulty copy of the gene, and the normal copy usually ensures normal function. However, if a male child inherits her faulty copy of the X chromosome, he will develop the condition, as he has no normal X chromosome (having inherited a Y chromosome from the father). Each male child of a woman who is a carrier of an X-linked recessive condition will have a 50% chance of inheriting it. Men with an X-linked condition cannot pass it on to their sons, but all their daughters will be carriers. X-linked recessive conditions include hemophilia, Duchenne muscular dystrophy, and fragile X.

Features of X-linked inheritance pattern (see *Figure 2.4*):
- more than one generation can be affected
- males are generally affected more severely than females in the family
- there is no evidence of male-to-male transmission

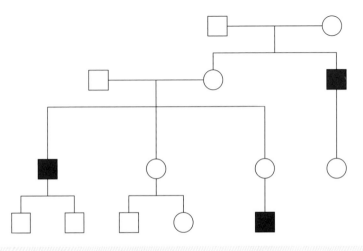

Figure 2.4. Typical X-linked pedigree pattern.

2.6 Making a numerical assessment of risk

When we refer to the possibility of a person developing a particular condition, or passing it onto their offspring, we are really talking about *chance*. However, in genetics this chance is generally known as the recurrence risk and so that is the term we will use here.

There is much evidence that people do not base their genetic decisions solely upon a numerical recurrence risk value. The individual's perception of the burden of the disease has a huge impact on their decision, and this is a very personal construct based on their own experience of the condition, what they have read or been told, and experience of similar situations. However, a numerical value may help the client, especially if their own assessment of the risk has been unrealistically high or low.

2.6.1 *Making a risk assessment based on inheritance pattern*

Using the data obtained from the family history and a knowledge of the inheritance pattern, the chance or recurrence risk can be calculated. This is fairly straightforward in some cases.

Case 1 – Autosomal dominant inheritance pattern

William has dominantly inherited adult polycystic kidney disease (APKD). This causes multiple cysts to develop in the kidneys, usually before the age of 30 years.

William and his wife are concerned about their two children, Kerry and Harry, and ask about the chance that Kerry and Harry will develop the condition. As William has one normal and one faulty copy of the gene for APKD, and only passes one copy of the gene into each sperm, each child was born with a 50% chance of inheriting the faulty gene. Any future children will also have a 50% chance of inheriting the condition (*Figure 2.5*).

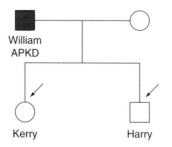

Figure 2.5. Pedigree of William's family.

Case 2 – Autosomal recessive inheritance pattern

Colin has a brother with cystic fibrosis, and he asks about his risk of being a carrier of the gene mutation (*Figure 2.6*).

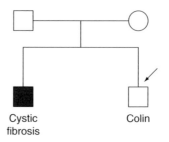

Cystic
fibrosis

Colin

Figure 2.6. Pedigree of Colin's family.

We know that Colin's brother inherited a faulty copy of the CFTR (cystic fibrosis transmembrane receptor) gene from both parents. Both Colin's parents are therefore carriers. Each time they had a child there were four possible combinations of **alleles**, as shown in *Figure 2.7*.

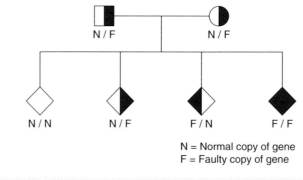

N = Normal copy of gene
F = Faulty copy of gene

Figure 2.7. Four possible outcomes from carrier parents.

However, Colin does not have cystic fibrosis, so we can eliminate the last possibility (F/F) from the calculation. There are three combinations remaining. In two of those combinations a faulty gene is passed on, therefore Colin's chance of being a carrier is two out of three, or a 2/3 chance.

Case 3 – X-linked recessive inheritance pattern

Ruth has two uncles, both of whom died with Duchenne muscular dystrophy. Because two of Ruth's uncles had the condition, we assume that her grandmother was a carrier, as it is unlikely for two new mutations to occur spontaneously in one family. Therefore Ruth's mother has a 50% risk of being a carrier; she had no sons (*Figure 2.8*).

Ruth's grandmother had two copies of the gene for DMD, one was faulty, the other normal. Ruth's mother was born at 50% risk of being a carrier. Ruth inherited only one copy of the gene from her mother, therefore her chance of being a carrier is 1 in 4 or 25%.

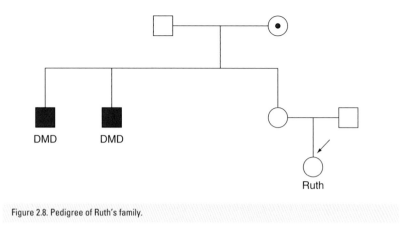

Figure 2.8. Pedigree of Ruth's family.

2.6.2 *Risk estimates based on empirical data*

There are many situations where the inheritance pattern is not as clear as in the examples given above. In some cases, the actual genetic basis of the condition is still not known, or the condition may be multi-factorial. Empirical data are then used to offer the family an idea of the level of risk.

Case 4 – Multi-factorial pattern

Josie and Fred have had a baby with bilateral renal agenesis (failure of development of the kidney). The baby has not survived. They are very concerned that they may have another child with this same condition (see *Figure 2.9*).

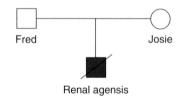

Figure 2.9. Pedigree of Josie and Fred's family.

Renal agenesis is not usually inherited as a **Mendelian** condition, but data show that about 5% of couples who have had one child with renal agenesis have another child with the same condition in a future pregnancy.

Josie and Fred are told that the risk of a fetus having renal agenesis in a future pregnancy is 5%.

2.7 **Bayesian calculations**

The Bayesian calculation is used in genetics for refining the recurrence risk for an individual. The theorem is attributed to Thomas Bayes, an eighteenth century nonconformist minister who was also said to be an excellent mathematician! The calculation enables us to take into account additional information that might alter the actual likelihood of the person being affected or being a carrier of a condition. Although the calculations may look complicated at first glance, if you just work through them step by step they are actually quite simple. However, unless you are involved in offering genetic counseling, you are unlikely to need to use these types of calculations. For the keen practitioner who would like to learn more, we have included instructions in *Appendix 1*.

2.8 Using the Hardy–Weinberg equation to calculate carrier risk

We have seen that it is possible to calculate carrier risk of a particular condition if there is a family history. However, sometimes it is necessary to calculate the population risk of carrying a particular genetic condition. This is the case when a person with no family history partners a carrier of a recessive condition. To calculate the risk to the offspring of this couple, the carrier risk of both partners is required. The Hardy–Weinberg equation of population genetics can be used for this purpose.

The equation states that:

$$p^2 + 2pq + q^2 = 1$$

where p is the normal allele and q is the mutated allele of a particular gene.

If q is the mutated recessive gene, then the frequency of carriers of the recessive gene is $2pq$. In reality, with a rare allele, the frequency of the normal allele (p) is regarded as 1. Therefore for practical purposes the carrier rate in the population (frequency of **heterozygotes**) is $2q$. Information about how to use this calculation is included in *Appendix 2*.

2.9 Lay knowledge and the perception of risk

Lay knowledge or lay belief are terms used to describe the information that exists in the family about the particular genetic condition that affects them. The beliefs are usually rooted in the family's experience of the condition, but may also be based upon general health beliefs, superstition or medical information previously passed on to them. Attributes that are unconnected to the genetic condition (such as hair color) may be linked to the experience of the disease, leading people in the family to believe, for example, that all the redheads in the family will get the condition. In other cases, the disease is linked to the sex of those affected, and if the only affected members of a family have all been male, the family may believe that only sons in the family are at risk.

As many people have only a sketchy idea of genetics, they may seek non-genetic explanations for what has happened in the family. Other information about influences on health may be used to draw conclusions about the cause of a disease or syndrome. For example, a mother who has a child with learning delay may question the quality of her diet during the pregnancy.

Application of lay knowledge will often lead to particular family members being identified as either being at high risk of the condition or likely to avoid it. This pre-selection of affected members can liberate from worry those who do not fit the criteria, but may place extra burdens on those who are predicted to be affected.

For genetic information to be useful for families, they must be able to fit any new information into their family story. It is helpful to use the family's own family tree when explaining the inheritance pattern, so that any discrepancies between the explanation and the lay knowledge held by that family can be addressed. If this is not done, the lay beliefs will persist, as the family's own experience is more powerful than an abstract scientific explanation. Family dynamics can be disrupted if the lay knowledge is challenged by new developments. The family may require time and support to adjust to a new way of thinking about the inheritance of the condition.

In taking decisions, the family will put weight on the burden of the disease as well as the chance of a family member being affected. If the burden of the disease is heavy, even a very low risk may seem oppressive. On the other hand, if the family views a disease as mild, they may consider any risk worth taking.

KEY PRACTICE POINT

When explaining an inheritance pattern to the family, use the family's own tree so that the family can integrate the information with their own family experience.

2.10 Conclusion

Drawing an accurate family tree is a skill that can be acquired through practice. The information in the family structure is the basis for risk estimation, but other relevant data can be used to refine the risk. However, risk estimation is only one component of genetic counseling and in the next chapter we will discuss counseling applications that may be used to support the client.

Further resources

www.geneticseducation.nhs.uk/family_history/Family_History_Series.pdf – National Genetics Education and Development Centre, Family history Series. *Guidance on taking family history and drawing pedigrees.*
www.hhs.gov/familyhistory/ – U.S. Surgeon General's Family History Initiative. *Draw your own pedigree online.*

Harper PS (2004) *Practical Genetic Counselling*, 6th Edition. London: Hodder Arnold. *Seminal text on genetic counseling, ideal reference work for any health setting.*

Test yourself

Q1. Practice drawing a family tree by doing your own.

Q2. Martin is the youngest of the three children in his family. He has two brothers. Martin has an uncle on his mother's side of the family who has β-thalassemia, an autosomal recessive condition. Martin's mother is younger than her affected brother and they have no other siblings. There are no other family members affected. Draw the pedigree of Martin's family. What is the chance that Martin is a carrier of the condition?

Q3. Bernice is 32 years old. Her paternal grandfather died at 47 years from an autosomal dominant form of hypertrophic cardiomyopathy. There is no history of cardiac problems in her father. What is Bernice's chance of developing the condition?

You learn Bernice's father died in a traffic accident at the age of 29 years. How does that change the way you discuss Bernice's risk with her?

Q4. Case discussion

Joyce attends a genetic clinic to talk about the family history of cancer. Joyce is a member of a large family with a known genetic mutation. When taking the family tree, the genetic counselor refers to the family tree she has in the notes and comments that the reason the genetics department knows that the gene is in the family is that samples have been looked at from Joyce's sister and her aunt who have had breast cancer. Joyce catches sight of the family tree upside down in the notes and asks why she is shaded in black like her sister and aunt. The counselor replies that it is because she had breast cancer. At this point Joyce becomes extremely angry and upset, demanding to know who told the genetics department that she had breast cancer; she had never been told she had breast cancer. It emerged that Joyce had had a breast reduction for cosmetic reasons and the family assumed that she had developed breast cancer. Joyce left the clinic still angry with the genetics team and her family and asked for a referral to another genetics centre.

How could this situation have been handled differently?

What does this example illustrate about reported family histories?

3 Counseling issues

3.1 Introduction to counseling in the context of genetic healthcare

Genetic counseling is primarily a communication process. In this chapter, the use of counseling skills to improve communication between professionals and families will be described. Several theories of counseling that could be useful when working with families will also be discussed.

First, it is important to differentiate between *using counseling skills*, and *active counseling*. In any healthcare interaction where the client has to consider a genetic risk, counseling skills are required. This obviously includes genetic counseling settings, but applies equally to a number of other situations that are far more common in healthcare settings.

Some example situations are as follows.
- A midwife offers a pregnant woman serum screening for **trisomy** 21 risk in the fetus.
- A practice nurse or general practitioner recommends a blood test for cholesterol levels in a person who has a family history of heart disease.
- A breast care nurse discusses routine mammography for screening in a woman with a family history of breast cancer.
- A surgical nurse discusses the benefits and risks of colonoscopy with a man who has a strong family history of colorectal cancer.
- A health visitor undertakes a developmental assessment in a child because of concerns about the child's delay in reaching milestones.

In each of these situations, the health professional is offering a test that could define the genetic status of the individual concerned (in the pregnant woman, this is of course the fetus). The result of the test may indicate an immediate health concern for that person, but may also give information about long-term concerns, the person's genetic status, and the risks to other members of the family. For example, if the man with a family history of bowel cancer is found to have multiple polyps in the sigmoid colon, he would be considered likely to have inherited a gene mutation for familial adenomatous polyposis (FAP), and the risk to his children of having the same condition is assessed as 50%. It is clear that these issues need to be discussed prior to testing, and the client's feelings about the potential results explored.

For this reason, counseling skills training for almost all health professionals is not only beneficial, but imperative. Many health professionals claim to be 'good communicators', but anecdotal reports from clients demonstrate that they often feel this is not the case. In one such case a woman gave birth to a baby with a cleft lip. The midwife kindly said to her 'It's such a pity, she would have been a lovely little girl'. This was probably meant to reassure the mother, but actually left her devastated. In another family, the general practitioner tried to reassure a mother about her son. The seven year old boy had recently been diagnosed with neurofibromatosis (NF). The doctor said that she shouldn't worry, because having NF was really no more problematic than having red hair, apparently forgetting that the boy's father had died from an osteosarcoma, directly linked with NF.

As clients are often in unfamiliar situations when they meet with health professionals, and may be anxious or concerned, skilful communication is essential if harm to the client is to be avoided. However, competence in healthcare is based on more than avoiding harm, and holistic healthcare involves enabling the client to voice their concerns and explore options.

3.2 The psychological needs of the client and the family

When working with any group of clients in a healthcare setting, the psychological needs of the client must be considered as part of the total package of care for that individual. When the client is facing genetic issues, the situation may be more complex because of the effect of the condition on more than one family member, possibly through many generations. There may be guilt at having passed a condition onto the children, blame towards sections of the family, or secrecy to try to hide the condition. Because being affected or at risk of a genetic condition can cause grief in many forms, clients may be in a state of perpetual mourning. For clients who experience this type of psychological pressure, counseling may provide an outlet for emotions that are hidden from the family.

Harding Family

Jennifer (nee Harding) is aged 44 years. Her father Cyril was affected with Huntington disease from the age of 50 years. Jennifer was only 18 when he was diagnosed. It was a huge shock to her; she had not known of the risk to her father or herself. Her father developed paranoia suddenly and was admitted to a psychiatric unit at the local hospital for 4 weeks. Even after he left hospital he was altered, and not the father she had known.

Jennifer had always wanted to be a nurse, but after her father became ill she couldn't face working in a hospital. She became a librarian.

When David proposed, she told him that she didn't feel she could risk having children. He knew her father and accepted this decision.

Jennifer dotes on her nieces and nephew. She is now almost too old to have her own family, but at times wonders if she has done the right thing, as her yearning for a child of her own is very strong. Cyril died at 62 years after becoming increasingly debilitated. Jennifer finds it so hard to visit her sister Mary, who is now affected, but feels guilty if she doesn't. She is sure Mary would not desert her if the situation was reversed.

Jennifer has lived with grief for many years. After the initial shock of her father's diagnosis, she lived with constant fear of his death. The diagnosis in her sister has awakened all the feelings of fear and distress she felt at the time her father was diagnosed. Jennifer asked whether prenatal testing would be possible if she became pregnant, and was referred to the genetic counselor. On meeting Jennifer to talk about possible prenatal diagnosis, the genetic counselor became aware of her mixed emotions, and made a contract with Jennifer to spend four sessions discussing these issues in a counseling environment.

When the counselor meets Jennifer, she identifies a number of areas of loss connected with the genetic condition in the family. Some of these are:

- *the loss of her father as a supportive parent*
- *the loss of her chosen career*
- *the loss of her confidence in her own future health*
- *the loss of the opportunity to have a family without undue concern*
- *the death of her father*
- *the loss of normal sibling relationships after the diagnosis in her sister*

3.3 Basic counseling skills

In any interaction between health workers and clients, it is obviously desirable that the client feels that their own concerns are heard and addressed, and that they have an opportunity to express feelings connected with their situation. The basic skills required to facilitate this are being able to:

- ask open questions
- reflect back the client's feelings in a way that affirms them
- paraphrase and summarize what the patient is saying to 'check you have the story right'
- interpret and use non-verbal communication
- be comfortable with silences

These tools of counseling will assist the practitioner to hear the client and give them the opportunity to discuss the issues with which they are most concerned. It is not possible to learn counseling via a textbook, as it is a very practical skill that requires both practice in a learning environment and a degree of self-awareness that can be developed within a learning group. However, it is possible to discuss some theories of counseling that may be useful in thinking about clients and the way in which health professionals may be able to support them in adapting to change.

3.4 Non-directiveness

The term non-directiveness has been the focus of much discussion in genetic counseling. It has emerged as a model for practice, partly as a reaction to the criticism that genetics has elements of eugenics. The client's choice is considered to be extremely important, and therefore the practitioner avoids directing the client. However, although in principle non-directiveness seems possible, in practice it has to be acknowledged that very few interactions in healthcare are completely without some form of guidance or direction. Pressure can be exerted in many ways, often subtly. It can be implied simply by the wording of certain choices (e.g. *'You can choose to terminate the pregnancy or you can keep your baby'*), or the amount of time spent discussing certain options.

A client may feel coerced into a decision if the counselor says that the majority of people make a particular decision, for example *'It is entirely your decision, but in my experience I find most people want to avoid having a child with Down syndrome'*.

However, the philosophy of non-directiveness does not mean that the counselor leaves the client unsupported in their efforts to make decisions. Facilitating the client in making their own informed decisions is an integral part of the role of a counselor, and requires a degree of skill. For this reason training in counseling skills is necessary. There are, of course, many situations in healthcare that require the use of counseling skills. While many professionals have a great deal of experience in communicating with clients, this is not always sufficient when giving genetic information. The use of the term genetic counselor has been controversial as a professional title because of the resistance of some practitioners to claiming counseling expertise. However, it is clear that in order to fulfil the definition of genetic counseling, skills in this area are required. Counseling skills are used within the session to:

■ enable and encourage the client to express their individual concerns
■ provide support to the client through the process of decision-making
■ help the client to adapt to living with the condition or to being at risk of a condition

3.5 Models of counseling

Counseling differs from the use of counseling skills, because in a counseling relationship both parties contract to meet for the purpose of exploring a psychological issue that is of concern to the client. The practitioner should be trained in counseling to the appropriate level, and should be receiving counseling supervision from an appropriately trained and experienced counselor.

There are many models of counseling that are appropriate for use in a genetic counseling setting. Those that are discussed here have been chosen because they can help the practitioner to interpret what is happening for the client, even in a single session. A model provides a framework for understanding the client's difficulties or behaviour, however, it is usually not appropriate to vocalize the explanation to the client in the session.

3.5.1 Person-centred counseling

Person-centred counseling was developed through the work of Carl Rogers[15], based on his belief that each person has the ability to solve their own problems and work through difficult situations using their own resources, providing that they have support from another person. The person-centred counselor is not 'an expert', who can solve the client's problems, but rather a supporter whose role is to reinforce the client's self-belief, and enable him or her to explore the situation in a safe emotional environment. Rogers devised the 'core conditions' for a positive counseling relationship: genuineness, empathy and warmth.

Genuineness. The counselor is real to him- or herself and to the client. To achieve this, the counselor requires a considerable degree of self-awareness and a belief in the equality of the client.

Empathy. One description of empathy is being able to 'walk in the other person's shoes'. Whereas sympathy involves feeling sorry for the other person, empathy is more connected with trying to understand how the client feels, and communicating that understanding.

Warmth. Understanding the client is not facilitative unless that can be conveyed. The 'gold standard' for the person-centred counselor is the ability to hold every person in unconditional positive regard. Whilst this is itself a challenge, it helps to reduce value judgements of the client and therefore increases the likelihood that the client will feel free to make the decision that is best for them.

A secondary group of core conditions are helpful in facilitating the client to explore his or her feelings and attitudes, but should only be used when an atmosphere of trust has been established between the client and counselor. These are immediacy, concreteness and challenge.

Immediacy. The use of immediacy in the session helps to reinforce the genuineness of the counselor, and to ground the session in the 'here and now'. The counselor notices and may comment on what is actually happening between the client and the counselor during the session. For example, the client may be clenching her fists, but saying *'I'm not angry'*. The counselor may bring this discrepancy to the client's attention by saying, *'You're saying you're not angry, but I notice that your fists are clenched'*. This helps the client to become aware of feelings that might be difficult to acknowledge, or of which they may not be consciously aware. Similarly, the client may use immediacy to comment on a client's reactions during the session. For example, the counselor is taking holiday leave, and tells the client that she will not be available for two weeks, then notices that the client has become withdrawn. The counselor may comment on this and use it to explore what her being away may mean for that client.

Challenge. Challenge is used when there are discrepancies in the client's account. It is not aggressive, but offered as a way of inviting the client to examine what is happening. For example, the client might say that she had always imagined herself as a mother, then say that it was lucky she didn't have children because she wouldn't have had time for them. This discrepancy in the story could be challenged to help the client become aware of her own feelings.

Concreteness. The counselor uses concreteness to maintain the reality of the discussion and help the client focus on what is currently relevant. For example, a man might be concerned about a diagnosis in his wife, but denies the impact of it on himself. The counselor needs to help him focus on the relevant issues.

Although young babies have a positive self-concept, the process of growing up inevitably damages that concept, and the person loses their confidence in their own ability to direct their lives. Through the use of the core conditions, the counselor aims to restore this positive self-concept, empowering the client. This is a fitting model for use in genetic counseling, where clients frequently have difficult decisions to make, and where the use of person-centred approach reinforces their ability to make those decisions.

3.5.2 Family systems theory

This model[16] is based on the theory that families work as systems, and changes in one area of the system have an effect on all other components. The system is greater than the sum of its parts, and usually adjusts to changes to function together coherently. However, if a change is not managed by the family, they may need help in 'reframing' what has happened to accommodate the change.

First-order change. When change occurs within a family, it may be first-order change that does not really alter the family arrangement. Family members maintain their relationships with one another in the same way.

Second-order change. Second-order change occurs when the family system really alters as a result of some intervening situation. The family needs to make an adjustment, if this is not possible in a constructive way, the family may need assistance to reframe their relationship, and assign different meanings to behaviour, feelings and relationships. Family therapy aims to help the family affect this change.

Family therapy is usually carried out by more than one counselor. One counselor may stay in the room with the family, while the other is observing from another room, via a two-way mirror. At some stage in the session the counselor will leave the room to discuss what is occurring with the observer. Some strategies that may be used to help the family to gain a new perspective are detailed below.

Reframing. This strategy involves putting a different perspective on the problem presented by the family. For example, a man who has early dementia is extremely moody. His wife finds it very difficult to cope and complains to the counselor that he is making her sick with worry. The husband's moody behavior may be expressed in terms of the wife's inability to deal with the behavior.

Positive connotation. Noble motivations and responses are ascribed to behavior, and negative labeling of clients is avoided. It is the intention rather than the actual behaviour that is relabeled. The wife's responses could be positively ascribed to her love for her husband and her wish for him to be more satisfied with life.

Metaphorical communication. Clients may be encouraged to use fantasy to describe their situation. Counselors may use metaphors to convey concepts, or ask the client to express their situation in sculpture, paintings, or models. One example could be asking the client to use different articles to represent family members, placing them in relation to each other.

Paradoxical directions. The person who is exhibiting the 'problem' behavior may be instructed to perform it at set times and places. For example, a child who overeats may be instructed to eat a particular food on the hour.

All of these strategies are used to try and help the family gain a new perspective on the situation and to regain homeostasis.

Harding Family

Jennifer's story – a family systems perspective

The family therapist might think about the changes that have occurred for Jennifer and her family. While Jennifer's sister's diagnosis does not on the surface seem to disrupt Jennifer's life, in reality it is a second-order change as it changes Jennifer's status in the family. She becomes a carer and, in addition, the family hopes rest on her as a survivor. The impact of her sister's diagnosis also makes her question her wish for children of her own.

3.5.3 *Psychodynamic theory*

Psychodynamic counselors use the client's past history to try to clarify current patterns of behavior[17]. This theory has its roots in Freudian theory, emphasizing the experience of the child as being of importance in establishing recurrent patterns of relating to others.

The relationship the client develops with the counselor is of importance to the therapeutic work. In providing an environment where the client feels valued and is encouraged to express his or her feelings, the counselor is said to model the 'good enough' parent. Thus the parent/child relationship can be re-experienced in a positive way, enabling the client to take responsibility for his or her own life choices.

As part of the therapeutic process, the counselor may draw parallels between the client/counselor relationship, current relationships for the client, and past relationships. This is called the triangle of insight. For example, a client who has difficulty establishing a close relationship with her disabled child may have lost an important person during childhood. The counselor may notice that the client is reluctant to commit herself to a contract with the counselor, fearing dependency. The counselor may interpret this behaviour as a recurring pattern of reluctance to become involved, due to fear of sudden loss of the person to whom the client has become attached.

Harding Family

Jennifer's story – the psychodynamic perspective

The psychodynamic counselor may interpret the relationship between Jennifer and herself as important because of Jennifer's loss of her father as a good enough parent during her growing years. The counselor may try to facilitate Jennifer in making her own choices, whilst offering her support, in the way a parent would do with an adolescent child.

The counselor might help Jennifer to relate her current distress about her sister to the fear she felt when her father was diagnosed (past history).

3.5.4 *Transactional analysis*

The transactional analysis (TA) model is based on the belief that all humans are born believing in their own worth and the worth of others, but that this belief often becomes damaged during childhood. The belief in your own self worth is called the *I'm okay* position, while belief in the worth of others is termed *you're okay*[18].

Therapeutic counseling is aimed at enhancing the client's belief in themselves, helping them to return to the 'I'm okay, you're okay' state that is necessary for healthy relating. Another aspect of the TA model is the use of the terminology *parent, adult, child*. The three ego states exist in each person, one being dominant at any particular moment in time. The parent ego state reinforces duty messages such as 'I should'. However, the parent state can also be expressed by behaving protectively towards others. The 'free' child is the more natural state, but the 'adapted' child may cause the individual to respond in a conforming way to 'parental' figures. The adult ego state influences the individual to consider the relative aspects of each course of action and pursues the most logical course.

TA can help to explain why we sometimes seemingly react irrationally to others. For example, a person who we find very dominant can evoke a reaction from our child state. The counselor may try to facilitate the client in responding from the adult state as far as possible. This means becoming aware of one's needs.

Harding Family

Jennifer's story – a transactional analysis perspective

The counselor might help Jennifer to appreciate that the guilt she feels that influences her decision to care for her sister comes from her 'parent' state (I should look after her). The desire to have a child may come from her child state, with strong input from the parent state about denying herself that wish. The counselor may work with Jennifer to help her decide what to do when in the adult mode.

3.6 Counseling supervision

Any professional who provides counseling support for clients should seek counseling supervision for their work. This is usually provided by an experienced counselor, who is not the person's line manager. The purpose of counseling supervision is to enable the counselor to explore and reflect on their own work with the client. In dealing with emotional areas, issues that impact on the counselor will inevitably emerge, and supervision helps to protect both the client and counselor from emotional harm.

In the UK, the Association of Genetic Nurses and Counsellors considered supervision such an important aspect of professional practice that they set up a Working Group which issued a report[19] that included the following definition of genetic counseling supervision:

> "Genetic counselling supervision is a formal and contractual arrangement, whereby genetic counsellors meet with a suitably trained and experienced supervisor to engage in purposeful, guided reflection of their work. Focusing on the dynamics between client and genetic counsellor, the aim of this process is to explore the inter-action between the counsellor and their client, and the impact of external factors on this, enabling counsellors to learn from experience, improve their practice and maintain competence. The overall intention is to enhance the quality and safety of client care and to promote the ongoing professional development of the genetic counsellor." (AGNC Supervision Working Group, 2007)

While those who work outside a clinical genetics service may feel such a formal process is inappropriate, the reason for counseling supervision is to ensure the psychological safety of both the client and counselor. It is therefore relevant for any health professional to consider the arrangements in place to facilitate safe practice. It is often possible to set up counseling supervision with a trusted and experienced colleague, if formal arrangements do not exist for supervision.

EXAMPLE OF COUNSELING SUPERVISION IN PRACTICE

Judy was a midwife counselor working in the antenatal clinic. She was on duty one morning when a woman came into the unit on her way to work because she had not felt fetal movements the previous day. She just "wanted to make sure everything was all right". Her husband was away for several days at a conference.

The fetal heartbeat was not seen on scan, and the woman was told her baby had died *in utero*.

Judy arranged to see the woman at home the following week for grief counseling.

When Judy was with the woman, she felt sad for her, but very angry with her husband. She felt unable to offer him any support.

In supervision, Judy puzzled over this, as she generally related well to both mothers and fathers. It was her supervisor who encouraged her to explore any personal issues that might have been influencing her attitude. She realized that she had been very angry with her father for not being present when her mother had died in hospital, and this feeling had been aroused by the circumstances of her patient. When she understood where the feelings had come from, she was able to relate to the bereaved father differently.

3.7 Conclusion

In all fields of healthcare, the use of counseling skills helps to enable the client to express themselves, and to make their own choices rather than respond to advice from others. Of course there are situations where healthcare advice is given appropriately, but in the area of genetics advice, giving is generally not appropriate. Training in counseling skills and ongoing counseling supervision are essential in enabling the professional to care for clients competently.

Further resources

www.geneticseducation.nhs.uk/tellingstories/ – Telling Stories – Understanding Real Life Genetics. *Website featuring the stories of families affected by genetic conditions, including the psychosocial impact of the condition.*

www.agnc.org.uk/About%20us/clinicalsupervision.htm – AGNC Counselling Supervision Report.

Egan G (1998) *The Skilled Helper*, 6th Edition. Pacific Grove: Brooks/Cole Publishing Company. *The how-to book of counseling skills.*

Evans C (2006) *Genetic Counselling: a Psychological Approach.* Cambridge: Cambridge University Press. *Counseling text specifically for genetic counselors.*

Hough M (2000) *A Practical Approach to Counselling.* Harlow: Longman. *A general text that presents a number of different counseling models and theories.*

Mearns D, Thorne B (1999) *Person-Centred Counselling in Action*, 2nd Edition. London: Sage Publications, Inc. *Counseling skills text based on Rogerian approach.*

Basic concepts in genetic science

4.1 Introduction

In the current scientific climate, it is difficult to believe that the double helical structure of DNA was only described as recently as 1953[20], and that the correct number of human chromosomes was finally identified in 1956[21]. During the course of only one generation, **karyotyping** became a commonplace method of diagnosis of chromosomal abnormalities, and DNA studies were being used to offer families reproductive choices previously denied to them. Since the 1980s, techniques in **cytogenetics** and **molecular genetics** have developed dramatically, adding to the information that is now accessible to families. As this new technology assumes more importance in everyday healthcare, the health professional has to have an understanding of its applications and limitations. With developments in genome sequencing and the findings from genome-wide association studies, the use of genetic technology is already moving from the confined area of medical genetics to almost every other speciality.

It is increasingly apparent that genetic factors influence many aspects of health. The influence of genes on health and disease could be thought of as a continuum. At one end of the spectrum are those conditions that are clearly caused by a **gene mutation**. This category includes conditions such as Huntington disease, Duchenne muscular dystrophy, and cystic fibrosis. At the other end are the diseases in which inborn genetic mutations do not appear to play a part. Environmental influences are thought to be far more relevant in the causation of diseases in this group, which could include lung cancer, and infectious diseases.

When functioning normally, a proportion of genes play an important role in protecting the body from disease. For example, the **tumor suppressor gene** *BRCA1* normally inhibits the overgrowth of cells in the breast tissue, therefore reducing the formation of tumors. It is only when these genes are faulty that the disease-inhibiting characteristics are lost. Thus it is not correct to say that a woman has a gene for breast cancer, but rather that she has a breast cancer gene mutation. The role of genes in cancer is discussed more fully in *Chapter 10*.

The aim of this chapter is to provide the health professional with basic scientific literacy to understand the practical application of genetics for families, as described in the rest of the book. This chapter begins with the larger units of genetic material that are visible with a light microscope (e.g. chromosomes), and moves on to smaller units (e.g. genes) that can only be analyzed using molecular genetic techniques. Before reading further, it might be helpful to refresh your memory of the key definitions below.

KEY DEFINITIONS

DNA: deoxyribonucleic acid. DNA is the biochemical substance which forms the human genome. It carries in coded form the information that directs the growth, development and function of physical and biochemical systems. It is usually present within the cell as two strands with a double helix confirmation (*Figure 4.1*). The strands consist of a backbone of sugars and are linked by paired bases. The bases in DNA are thymine (T), adenine (A), cytosine (C) and guanine (G). T and A will always pair, as will C and G, and it is this pairing that allows for replication of the DNA. The order of the bases specifies the sequence of amino acids, which are the building blocks of proteins. Each amino acid is coded for by a specific sequence of three bases (**codon**).

Gene: the fundamental physical and functional unit of heredity consisting of a sequence of DNA. Our genes direct the growth, development and function of every part of our physical and biochemical systems and are the unit by which these characteristics are passed from generation to generation. Genes consist of coding sequences (**exons**) and non-coding sequences (**introns**).

Chromosomes: the physical structures into which the DNA is packaged within the nucleus of cells (*Figure 4.2*). The usual number of chromosomes in humans is 46, normally found as 23 pairs. Pairs numbered 1 to 22 are identical in males and females. In addition, females have two identical X chromosomes, and males have an X chromosome and a Y chromosome.

4.2 The chromosomes

4.2.1 Mitosis and meiosis

The chromosomes are packages of genetic material, stored within the nucleus of each cell. Almost every human cell is **diploid,** which means that they contain two copies of each of the **autosomes** (chromosomes 1–22), and two sex chromosomes. The exceptions to this are, of course, the germ cells (ova and sperm) in which there is only one copy of each chromosome – these cells are described as **haploid.** Throughout the human lifetime, cells are produced for new growth or to replace dead cells. Diploid cells are produced by the process of **mitosis** (*Figure 4.3*).

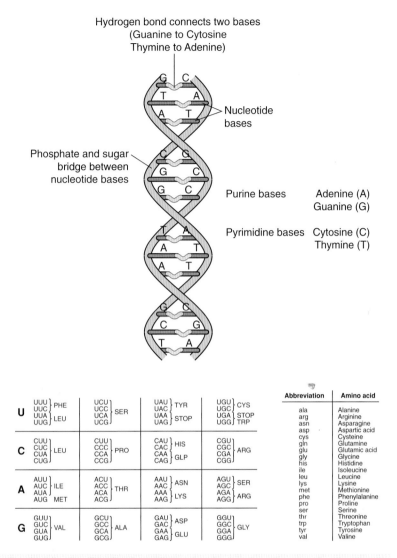

Figure 4.1. The DNA molecule and list of codons.

Within the ovary or testis, haploid cells are made by a different process, called **meiosis** (*Figure 4.4*).

In the first part of the meiotic cycle (meiosis 1), after DNA replication the chromosomes pair up and exchange material in a process called **recombination**. One of each pair of the chromosomes migrates to the opposite end of the cell before the cell divides into two daughter cells, each with 23 single chromosomes. During the second meiotic division in these two daughter cells, the two **chromatids** of each chromosome separate resulting in four daughter cells, each containing only one of each pair of chromosomes. If an error occurs during the **disjunction** of the two chromatids, then the resultant **gamete** may contain an abnormal number of chromosomes (*Figures 4.5* and *4.6*).

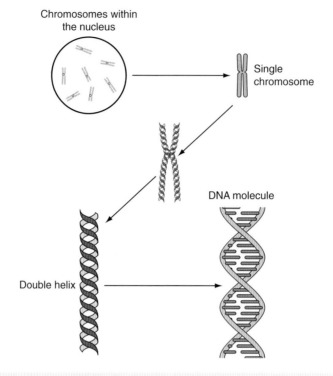

Chromosomes within
the nucleus

Single
chromosome

DNA molecule

Double helix

Figure 4.2. Relationship between a chromosome and DNA molecule.

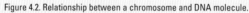

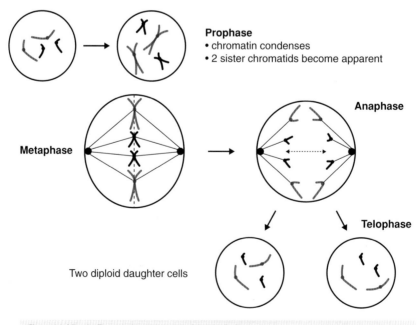

Prophase
• chromatin condenses
• 2 sister chromatids become apparent

Metaphase

Anaphase

Telophase

Two diploid daughter cells

Figure 4.3. Mitosis. Figure redrawn from an original by Dr Simon Holden.

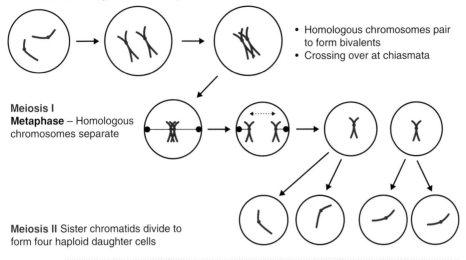

Meiosis I Prophase – DNA replicates to form sister chromatids

- Homologous chromosomes pair to form bivalents
- Crossing over at chiasmata

Meiosis I Metaphase – Homologous chromosomes separate

Meiosis II Sister chromatids divide to form four haploid daughter cells

Figure 4.4. Meiosis. Figure redrawn from an original by Dr Simon Holden.

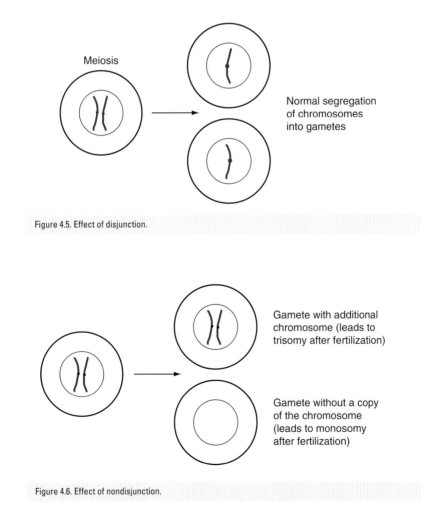

Meiosis

Normal segregation of chromosomes into gametes

Figure 4.5. Effect of disjunction.

Gamete with additional chromosome (leads to trisomy after fertilization)

Gamete without a copy of the chromosome (leads to monosomy after fertilization)

Figure 4.6. Effect of nondisjunction.

4.2.2 *Chromosomal inheritance*

Meiosis differs from mitosis in two important aspects. The first and obvious difference is the resultant numbers of chromosomes in the daughter cell. This is, of course, necessary to ensure that the embryo contains only two copies of each chromosome. The second difference is a result of recombination (*Figure 4.7*).

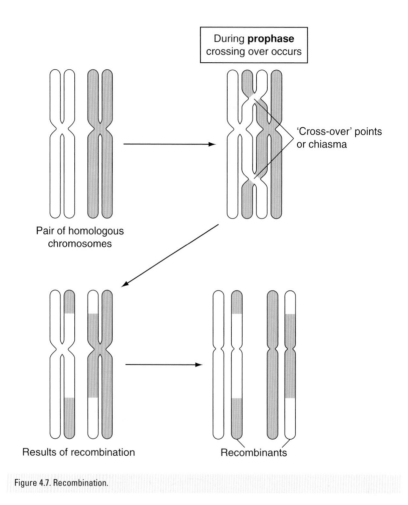

During **prophase** crossing over occurs

'Cross-over' points or chiasma

Pair of homologous chromosomes

Results of recombination

Recombinants

Figure 4.7. Recombination.

During the first meiotic division, each pair of chromatids is connected at junctions called **chiasmata** (the singular is *chiasma*). The chromosome inherited by that individual from their mother is linked with the chromosome inherited from the father. There is some exchange of the chromosomal material between the **homologous pairs**, such that the resultant two chromatids are a combination of maternal and paternal chromosomes.

The numbers of different combinations are vast, and this phenomenon therefore results in each child being a unique combination of genes derived from all four grandparents. As already stated, the normal number of chromosomes within a human **somatic** cell is 46. However, the chromosomal arrangement can differ in a number of significant ways that may have implications for the health and development of the person concerned.

In some cases, an individual may have two or more different chromosome arrangements (see *Table 4.1*), with one arrangement present in some cells, and a different one in other cells in the body. For example, a child may have trisomy 18 in some cells and a normal chromosome arrangement in others (karyotype 46,XY/47,XY,+18). This is called **mosaicism**. Individuals with a mosaic form of a chromosomal condition generally have a less severe phenotype than those with 100% of cells with the abnormality. Placental mosaicism is also possible and the abnormal karyotype may be restricted to the placenta.

Table 1 Classification of chromosomal rearrangements.

Chromosomal rearrangement	Clinical examples
Changes to the total number of chromosomes (aneuploidy)	
Trisomy	Trisomy 21 – Down syndrome Trisomy 18 – Edwards syndrome Trisomy 13 – Patau syndrome
Monosomy	Partial **monosomy** of autosomes may occur, but complete monosomy of any autosome would not be compatible with life. Cri du chat syndrome is an example of partial monosomy (4p −)
Sex chromosome **aneuploidy**	Turner syndrome 45,X Klinefelter syndrome 47,XXY
Robertsonian translocation	Robertsonian translocation (*Figure 4.8*) of chromosomes 14 and 15, or 14 and 21 is relatively common
Changes in the structure of specific chromosomes	
Balanced reciprocal translocation (*Figure 4.9*)	There may be an exchange of chromosomal material between any two chromosomes
Deletion	Microdeletion of 22q causes velocardiofacial syndrome
Duplication	Can occur in any chromosome
Insertion (*Figure 4.10*)	Can occur in any chromosome
Inversion: paracentric (*Figure 4.11* or pericentric (*Figure 4.12*)	Can occur in any chromosome

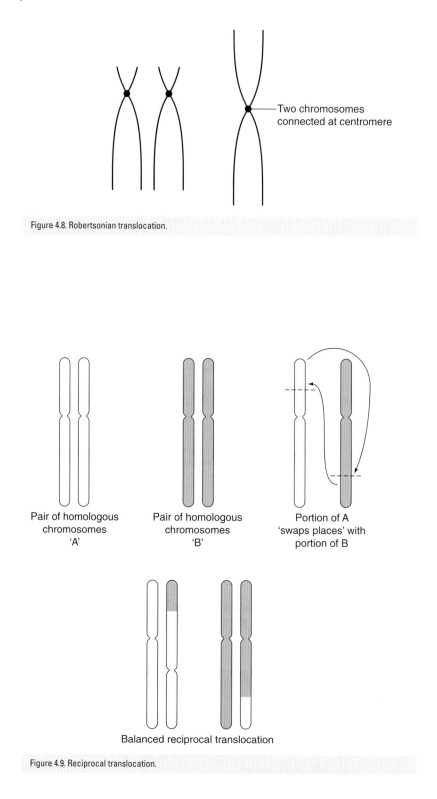

Figure 4.8. Robertsonian translocation.

Two chromosomes connected at centromere

Pair of homologous chromosomes 'A'

Pair of homologous chromosomes 'B'

Portion of A 'swaps places' with portion of B

Balanced reciprocal translocation

Figure 4.9. Reciprocal translocation.

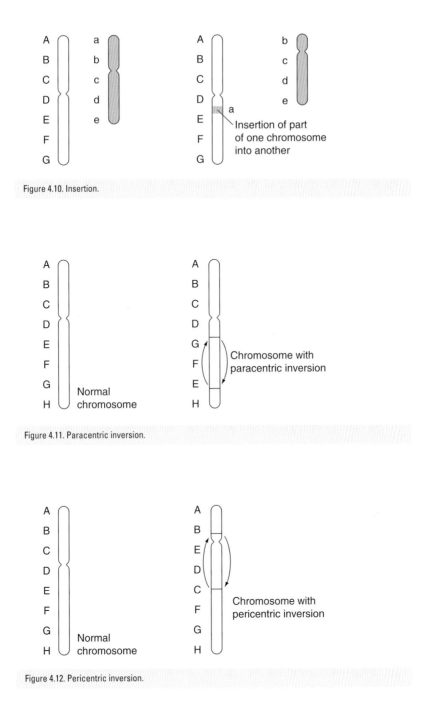

Figure 4.10. Insertion.

Insertion of part of one chromosome into another

Figure 4.11. Paracentric inversion.

Chromosome with paracentric inversion

Normal chromosome

Figure 4.12. Pericentric inversion.

Chromosome with pericentric inversion

Normal chromosome

KEY PRACTICE POINT

The results of a karyotype performed on the chorionic villi that show a chromosome abnormality in some placental cells should be checked to ascertain if the fetal cells have the same karyotype.

New techniques of molecular analysis such as **comparative genome hybridization** (CGH, described in *Section 4.4.2*) will detect very small areas of the genome where there are **deletions** or **duplications** (copy number variation). Some of these copy number variations may be significant, others will not. It is possible that in the future CGH will replace traditional visual examination of the chromosomes using a light microscope[22].

It used to be said that as a general heuristic, changes in the *balance* of the chromosomal material would have serious implications for the intellectual and physical development of the individual. However, as the ability to detect smaller changes increases, it is clear that it is possible to detect imbalances that may have no clinical significance.

4.2.3 *Imprinting*

In some areas of the genetic material, the maternally and paternally derived copies are expressed differently. **Imprinting** is said to occur if the copy from the parent of a particular sex is 'switched off'. For example, the genes that are implicated in Prader–Willi syndrome (PWS) and Angelman syndrome (AS) are located close to each other on chromosome 15. The maternal copy of the gene is switched off or imprinted in the PWS region. If a child has no working copy of this gene from the father, they will develop PWS. Similarly, the paternal copy is imprinted in the AS region, and therefore a child requires a copy of the gene from the mother or they will develop AS.

4.2.4 *Uniparental disomy*

In some circumstances, a child may accidentally inherit two copies of a region of the chromosomal material from one parent. This may apply to a full or partial chromosome. If the uniparental disomy (UPD) includes an imprinted region, then a genetic condition may result from the lack of genetic instruction from the relevant parent.

Possible mechanism underlying UPD. During meiosis, a non-disjunction event might result in the ovum or sperm having two copies of a particular chromosome. After fertilization, the trisomy may be corrected by the loss of one copy of that particular chromosome. However, if the copy that is lost comes from the parent that contributed only one copy, the two remaining copies will have originated from the same parent. This will result in UPD and is called trisomy rescue (*Figure 4.13*).

4.3 Investigating the chromosome structure

4.3.1 *Karyotyping*

It is possible for diagnostic purposes to study the chromosome structure of an individual or fetus. In most cases, this is done in a genetics laboratory by a

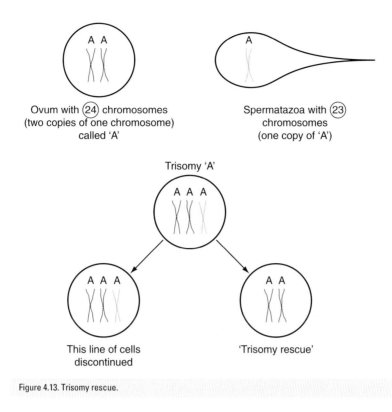

Figure 4.13. Trisomy rescue.

trained cytogeneticist. The chromosome structure is not easily seen during interphase, so cells are cultured in a tissue medium so they can be studied during mitotic division. When sufficient numbers of cells are undergoing metaphase, the process is 'frozen' by adding an agent such as colchicine (*Figure 4.14*). This effectively destroys the spindle fibers and the next stage of mitosis (anaphase) is not reached. Without the supporting spindle fibers, the chromosomes spread more evenly around the cell nucleus. A salt solution is

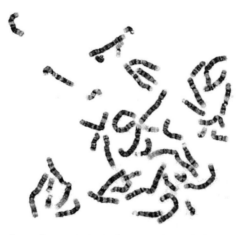

Figure 4.14. Metaphase spread.

added to the preparation to swell the cells, further separating the chromosomes and enabling them to be viewed more easily by the cytogeneticist. The chromosome preparation is 'fixed', placed on a slide, and viewed under the microscope.

A trained cytogeneticist is able to differentiate between the different chromosomes, assessing not only the total number but also the length and structural normality of each chromosome. The use of staining techniques (such as **G-banding**) assists in the differentiation of each part of the chromosome, so that disruptions to the normal arrangement can be detected more easily (*Figure 4.15*).

It is possible for diagnostic purposes to study the constitutional karyotype, in situations such as the following:

1. after a couple has had several spontaneous abortions, to detect a possible balanced translocation in one of the parents

2. when an unbalanced arrangement is suspected in a child who has learning difficulties and/or dysmorphic features

3. during pregnancy, when fetal cells are obtained via amniocentesis or chorionic villus sampling (also called chorionic villus biopsy)

Chromosome studies can be performed on a variety of tissues. Lymphocytes from a venous blood sample are usually the cells of choice. They are easily obtainable, grow readily in cell culture medium, and provide a good quality chromosome preparation for study. Cells from skin or other tissues (e.g. from a fetus following **stillbirth**) can also be used. For the purposes of prenatal diagnosis, cells from the chorion or fetal skin cells are used for the culture. Prenatal diagnosis is discussed in detail in *Chapter 7*. Due to the requirement to culture the tissues, in many cases the karyotype result will not be available for up to 7 days. The exception is the direct examination of cells from the

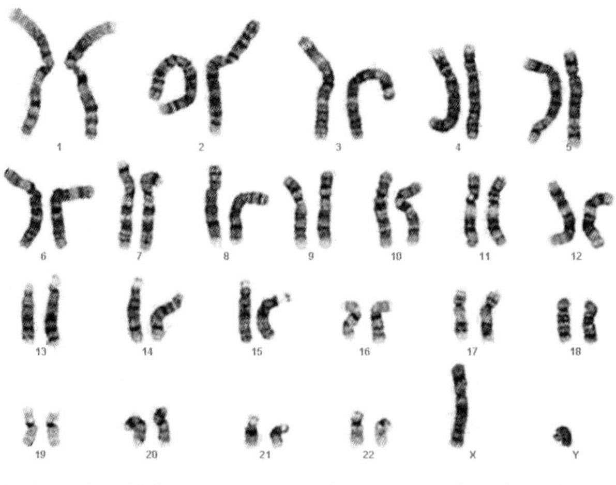

Figure 4.15. G-banded karyotype.

chorionic villus. Where a rapid result is needed for clinical purposes (e.g. for a sick neonate), a less detailed result can be made available more quickly.

Chromosome studies may also be requested to aid classification and management of some cancers, for example, chronic myeloid leukemia. In this situation the chromosome abnormality will have arisen in the bone marrow as part of the disease process. It is somatic rather than constitutional.

4.3.2 *Chromosomal nomenclature*

When reporting the results of a traditional karyotype, the cytogeneticist will always use a standard (ISCN – International System for Cytogenetic Nomenclature) nomenclature . The short arm of each chromosome is termed the 'p' arm (for petit) and the long arm is labelled 'q'. A report will include the following details:

- the total number of chromosomes observed
- the type and number of sex chromosomes
- any anomaly or abnormality of the chromosomes – a deletion is denoted by a 'subtraction' sign and any additional material is preceded by an 'addition' sign

Using this method, a normal male karyotype will be written as 46,XY and the normal female as 46,XX.

The karyotype of a male child with Down syndrome due to the presence of an additional chromosome will be reported as 47,XY,+21, denoting that the additional chromosome is identified as chromosome 21 (*Figure 4.16*).

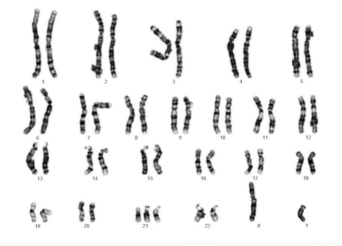

Figure 4.16. Karyotype of a male child with Down syndrome. Photograph supplied by the Cytogenetics Laboratory, Southmead Hospital, Bristol.

A female child with cri-du-chat syndrome will have a karyotype reported as 46,XX,5p− (*Figure 4.17*).

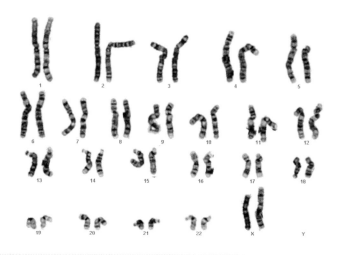

Figure 4.17. Karyotype of a female child with cri-du-chat syndrome. Photograph supplied by the Cytogenetics Laboratory, Southmead Hospital, Bristol.

4.4 Molecular cytogenetics

Increasingly, techniques involving molecular analysis or analysis of the DNA are used to investigate chromosome structure. The division that used to exist between molecular genetics and cytogenetics is becoming increasingly blurred. This is a rapidly moving area of technological development and a few current examples will be given.

4.4.1 *Fluorescence* in situ *hybridization*

Fluorescence *in situ* hybridization **(FISH)** is a technique (*Figure 4.18*) used in the laboratory to detect very small deletions or rearrangements in a chromosome. It is a test that is performed when a specific microdeletion or rearrangement is suspected by the clinician.

A **probe** (i.e. a small sequence of DNA) that matches the normal DNA sequence on the portion of the chromosome to be studied is attached to a fluorescent marker. When the probe is mixed with the chromosome preparation, it adheres to the normal chromosome(s), producing a colored signal. If an autosomal deletion is present, only one signal will be observed, as the probe will be unable to attach itself to the abnormal chromosome. Rearrangements can also be detected if the signal is not where it is expected to be. This technique is frequently used to test for the microdeletion of chromosome 22, known to cause velocardiofacial (or Di George) syndrome.

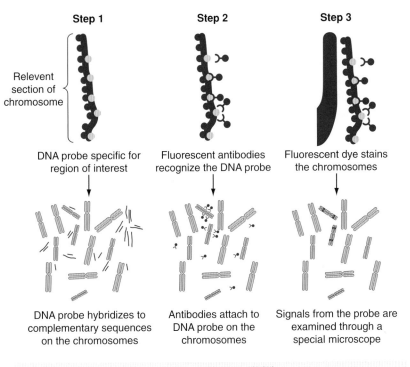

Step 1

Step 2

Step 3

Relevent section of chromosome

DNA probe specific for region of interest

Fluorescent antibodies recognize the DNA probe

Fluorescent dye stains the chromosomes

DNA probe hybridizes to complementary sequences on the chromosomes

Antibodies attach to DNA probe on the chromosomes

Signals from the probe are examined through a special microscope

Figure 4.18. Technique used in fluorescence *in situ* hybridization (FISH).

4.4.2 *Comparative genome hybridization*

By applying molecular methods of analysis, it is possible to examine the whole genome looking for variation in the number of copies of particular areas of the DNA which will show very small deletions or duplications of the chromosomes. These are sometimes called copy number variations. In a similar way to FISH, DNA from the patients and from a normal control is labeled with different colors and mixed. This mixture is then **hybridized** to normal metaphase chromosomes or, for array CGH, to a slide containing hundreds or thousands of defined DNA probes. The ratio of the fluorescence or color is used to determine regions of DNA gain or loss in the patient. Some of these areas of gain or loss may have no significance, while others will be significant. Follow-up investigations may be required including checking other members of the family or searching databases of previously described findings to determine the significance of the results. It is possible that in the future these techniques may replace karyotyping for identifying duplications and deletions of chromosome material. As the methods for looking for imbalances of chromosomes or DNA become more detailed, they also become much more difficult to both interpret and explain to families. The clinician needs to have regular contact with the laboratory scientists and other clinical colleagues in order to help the families understand the implications of the molecular findings.

4.5 Mendelian inheritance

Gregor Mendel, an Augustine monk, solved the riddle of the unit of heredity around the same time as Darwin was developing his theory of evolution. Mendel's experiments showed that inherited traits are not caused by blending of the characteristics of previous generations but by the inheritance of distinct units of heredity, which we now know as genes. The inheritance patterns in a family tree that are caused by single genes are known as **Mendelian**.

Mendel's experiments were done with plants. He discovered that if he crossed short and tall pea plants all the offspring were tall (*Figure 4.19*). He described tall stature as dominant over short stature. He then crossed these tall plants and discovered that about a quarter of their offspring were short. The hidden **recessive** gene for shortness was being expressed. He established that genes come in pairs and that if one characteristic is dominant and the other is recessive, the recessive characteristic will not be expressed unless both members of the pair of genes are recessive. This discovery was made many years before the actual discovery of DNA.

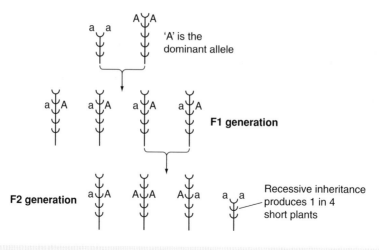

Figure 4.19. Second generation cross of short and tall peas.

In a species, the single gene responsible for a trait such as stature occupies the same position or **locus** on a chromosome. Each single copy of the gene at the same locus is termed an allele. One copy or allele is inherited from each parent. Within the human population it is possible for there to be many different alleles or versions of the gene at one locus. Within a normal individual there will be a maximum of two different alleles at any one locus. This is because each individual has a maximum of two copies of each gene. This concept will become important to understand when we discuss **linkage** later on in the chapter. These different alleles are simply variations of a normal DNA sequence and they need not be mutations within genes. If an animal or plant carries two identical alleles at a locus they are said to be **homozygous;** if they carry two different alleles at a locus they are **heterozygous.**

One way of describing the concept of alleles to a client is to use a box of colored balls containing at least two of each color. If they choose two balls they may have two of the same color or two differently colored balls. Selecting two balls of the same color represents homozygosity, whereas the different colored balls represent heterozygosity.

In human genetics there are theoretically five patterns of Mendelian inheritance. In practice, only three of these patterns are encountered frequently. These have been described in *Chapter 2*.

4.6 Expression and penetrance

The DNA sequence in the gene does not code for a protein directly. The code acts as a template for the production of **messenger RNA** (ribonucleic acid). The mRNA leaves the nucleus and binds to ribosomes where it directs the production of proteins. The string of amino acids is built up as each three-base sequence in the mRNA codes for one amino acid (*Figure 4.20*). The actual

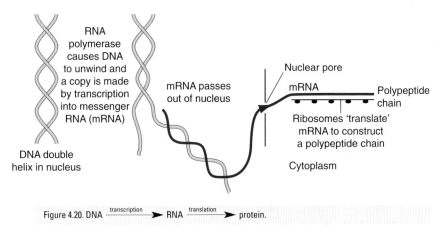

Figure 4.20. DNA $\xrightarrow{\text{transcription}}$ RNA $\xrightarrow{\text{translation}}$ protein.

physiologically active protein, for example, hemoglobin, may depend upon the action of several genes (*Figure 4.21*). Although every cell in the body with a nucleus has the same genetic code, not all the genes in every cell are switched on. The genes that are expressed at any one time will depend on the stage of development of the organism and the function of the cell.

A gene mutation may not always be obvious within a family tree because it is not fully **penetrant**. When the family tree is taken it may reveal individuals who must have inherited the gene but who do not manifest the condition.

The inheritance pattern of most of the high-risk cancer gene mutations is autosomal dominant, but they show reduced **penetrance**. Whilst a predisposition for cancer is inherited, some people who inherit a predisposition for cancer will not go on to develop the disease. If a person dies of an unrelated condition before the signs and symptoms of a late onset genetic

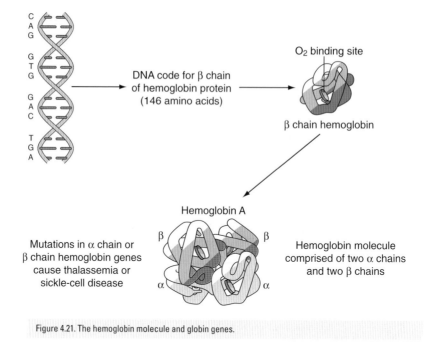

Figure 4.21. The hemoglobin molecule and globin genes.

disease occur, then the gene will appear to 'skip' a generation. The real explanation may be that the gene is only fully penetrant by old age.

Another explanation for a gene mutation not being obvious within a family tree is variable **expression** at the cellular level. A specific mutation may cause a wide variety of signs and symptoms, even within the same family. This is often most obvious in conditions which affect a number of different body systems, e.g. Marfan syndrome. Some family members who have the gene have serious complications such as dislocated membranes and a dilated aortic root. Other family members are simply tall and have hyperflexible joints. For this reason a careful clinical examination is necessary before someone is considered not to be at risk.

The possibility of variable expression and/or reduced penetrance of a condition should always be taken into account when taking a family history, to ensure all family members who are at risk are detected.

4.7 Genetic mutations

4.7.1 Types of mutations

Point mutations. Any change in the sequence of DNA within a gene is a mutation in that gene. Many mutations are harmless, either because they occur in the non-coding portion of the gene or because they make no difference to the eventual amino acid sequence. Alterations of a single base are called **point mutations.**

The type of disruption in the sequence of the DNA caused by point mutations. As discussed in previous sections, the DNA code is read in sequences of three bases, each three-base codon coding for a single amino acid.

CGGGTTTTGAAGCCGGGC

CGG	GTT	TTG	AAG	CCG	GGC
Arg	Val	Leu	Lys	Pro	Gly

To illustrate the point we will use a simple well-known sentence.

The Cat Sat On* The Mat

(NB On* is used to simply give all words three components.)

If there is a change in one of the letters the way the sentence reads is affected in different ways depending on what the change is. A point mutation would be the substitution of one letter for another, e.g.

The	Cat	Sat	On*	The	Rat
CGG	GTT	TTG	AAG	CCG	AGC
Arg	Val	Leu	Lys	Pro	Ser

This change still allows the sentence to be read although the sense is changed slightly. This would be equivalent to a **missense** point mutation. It may or may not cause a disruption to the final protein structure. Most proteins can tolerate some change to their amino acid sequence.

The	Cat	Smt	On*	The	Mat
CGG	GTT	TAG	AAG	CCG	GGC
Arg	Val	**STOP**			

This change has disrupted the sense of the sentence and would be equivalent to a **nonsense** mutation. Nonsense mutations cause the translation of the mRNA to end prematurely, resulting in a shortened protein. In most cases this happens because the mutation causes the codon to be read as a **stop codon.** Nonsense mutations usually have a serious effect on the encoded protein and may cause a mutant phenotype.

Insertion or deletion of one or more bases may also cause mutant phenotypes. The effect of these depends on whether the number of bases involved is a multiple of three or not. If it is a multiple of three the reading frame of the DNA sequence remains constant although there will be extra or missing amino acids. The exact phenotypic effects of these **in frame** mutations will depend on the effect of the mutation on the structure of the encoded protein.

The	Sat	On*	The	Mat		
CGG	TTG	AAG	CCG	GGC		
The	**Fat**	Cat	Sat	On*	The	Mat
CGG	**GGT**	GTT	TTG	AAG	CCG	GGC

If the number of bases inserted or deleted are not multiples of three then the reading frame is disrupted and the sequence of amino acids downstream from the mutation will be read differently. These **frameshift** mutations usually have a serious effect on the eventual protein.

The	CaS	atO	n*T	heM	at	
CGG	GTT	TGA	AGC	CGG	GC	
Tth	eCa	tSa	tOn	*Th	eMa	t
CCG	GGT	TTT	GAA	GCC	GGG	C

Mutations that have no effect on the encoded protein and therefore do not result in a mutant phenotype, or that occur in the non-coding portion of the genome, are called **polymorphisms**. They tend to accumulate in the DNA of organisms and contribute to the variability between individuals.

Gross mutations. Large sections of DNA can also be altered and these mutations normally disrupt the amino acid sequence. Deletions are a loss of a portion of DNA which may just be part of the gene or the entire gene sequence. There may be sequences of DNA inserted either from another portion of the genome or as **duplications**. A novel mutation responsible for a number of human diseases such as Huntington disease and fragile X syndrome is an **expansion** of triplet repeats. Some portions of the genome consist of a series of repeats of bases. An expansion of the normal number of repeats can cause a mutant phenotype.

Normal sequence

CGGGTTCAGCAGCAGAAGCCGGGC

Mutant expanded sequence

CGGGTTCAGCAGCAGCAGCAGCAGCAGCAGCAGAAGCCGGGC

It is important to remember that although genetic mutations can cause human disease, random mutations have contributed to the development of the myriad species on the earth today.

4.7.2 Molecular tests

Molecular genetic laboratories use a variety of different techniques to detect mutations or to track genes through families. The current basis of much genetic testing in clinical genetics is the **polymerase chain reaction (PCR)**. With PCR, specific DNA sequences can be copied many times to yield large quantities of the particular portion of DNA corresponding to genes or fragments of genes. These can then be analyzed or manipulated. The exact method of analysis used will depend upon the characteristics of the DNA sequence of interest and the type of potential mutations. The technique of PCR has also been important in the development of forensic DNA analysis. It has allowed the amplification of small amounts of DNA to provide a unique DNA fingerprint, which can be used as evidence.

Polymerase chain reaction. Amplification of the target DNA sequence occurs through repeated cycles of DNA synthesis. In clinical genetics the usual source of the DNA template used for the reaction is DNA extracted from cells from a patient. As in karyotyping, this can be any nucleated cell and a blood sample is commonly used. DNA can also easily be extracted from cells in the saliva or scraped from the inside of the cheek (buccal smear). This technique can also be used for prenatal diagnosis. Although DNA analysis is possible on cells harvested from amniotic fluid, the preferred sample is a chorionic villus biopsy, as this will yield greater amounts of DNA.

In addition to the target DNA, the other components of a PCR are:
- the primers – short sequences of single-stranded DNA that bind by complementary **base pairing** either side of the sequence containing the gene of interest
- DNA polymerase – an enzyme that copies the target sequence and that acts at a specific temperature
- molecules corresponding to the four bases – these are used in the synthesis of new DNA strands

In a PCR (*Figure 4.22*), the template DNA (usually all the chromosomal DNA) is put in solution with the primers, the DNA polymerase and the bases. The

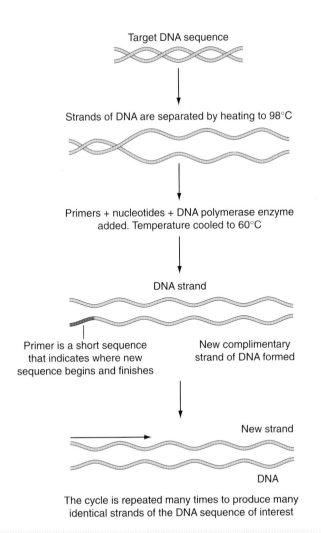

Target DNA sequence

↓

Strands of DNA are separated by heating to 98°C

↓

Primers + nucleotides + DNA polymerase enzyme added. Temperature cooled to 60°C

↓

DNA strand

Primer is a short sequence that indicates where new sequence begins and finishes

New complimentary strand of DNA formed

↓

New strand

DNA

The cycle is repeated many times to produce many identical strands of the DNA sequence of interest

Figure 4.22. PCR.

reaction is heated to destabilize the double helical structure of the template DNA, which then separates into two single strands (denaturing). The reaction is then cooled to a temperature that allows the primers to bind to the single-stranded DNA without allowing the double helix to reform (annealing). It is then heated to the temperature that allows the DNA polymerase to become active. The polymerase copies the sequence of the template DNA, starting at the primers and using the bases present in the reaction for synthesis of new single DNA strands (synthesis).

This cycle is repeated 20–40 times depending on how much of the target sequence was present in the original DNA template. In the first cycle synthesis carries on beyond the end of the target sequence because there is nothing to stop it. Over subsequent cycles, the newly synthesized strands, which end with a primer sequence themselves, act as templates and eventually only the target sequence is amplified.

Once sufficient target DNA has been generated, it can be used for clinical analysis or research. The techniques used to identify specific known gene mutations depend on the nature of the mutation. Analysis of specific mutations often utilizes DNA probes that hybridize to the mutation. DNA probes are single-stranded specific DNA sequences that have been radioactively or fluorescently labeled. If a probe is specific for a mutation then it will show a signal if the mutation is present and will not show a signal if it is absent. Probes may be designed to detect either normal or mutated sequences.

Quantitative PCR (QfPCR). By attaching a fluorescent probe to the area of interest it is possible to measure the amount of PCR product (*Figure 4.23*). By comparing it to a control sample, excess or reduced amounts can be detected. This can be used to detect known deletions, for example, in DMD carriers. It can also be used as a quick test to detect extra numbers of chromosomes, for example, when trisomy 21, 13, or 18 are suspected. QfPCR is now used in some areas instead of full karyotyping as the diagnostic test when screening for Down syndrome. This will be discussed in more detail in *Chapter 7*.

Linkage studies. For some genetic diseases, the mutant phenotype can be caused by a variety of different mutations in the same gene. If the exact mutation is not known, genetic testing with a family may be possible using linkage studies. Linkage testing depends upon the fact that there is considerable variation in the human genome between individuals and between homologous chromosomes within individuals. Molecular genetic techniques are being continuously developed utilizing this variability for the analysis of genes and for examining differences between individuals.

Linkage is the tendency for alleles whose loci are located close to each other to be passed on together on the same chromosome (*Figure 4.24*). The closer together on a chromosome the alleles are, the more likely they are to be inherited together. If alleles are further apart on a chromosome then, because

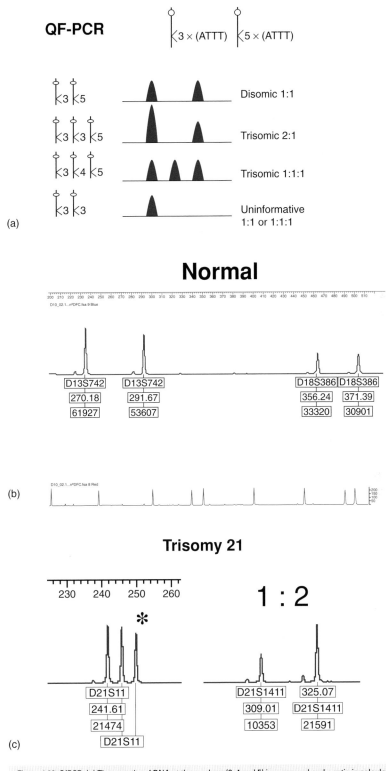

Figure 4.23. QfPCR. (a) The quantity of DNA at the markers (3, 4 and 5) is measured and a ratio is calculated. (b) The markers for chromosome 13 (D13S742) and chromosome 18 (D18S386) are disomic and in a ratio of 1:1 therefore normal. (c) The marker for chromosome 21 (D21S11) is trisomic. The other marker for chromosome 21 (D21S1411) is in a ratio of 2:1 Therefore there is trisomy 21.

of recombination during meiosis, the chance of them being inherited together
is reduced (see *Section 4.2.2* and *Figure 4.7*).

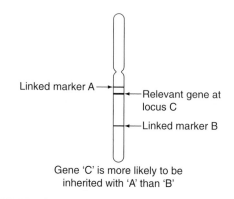

Gene 'C' is more likely to be
inherited with 'A' than 'B'

Figure 4.24. Linkage.

The phenomenon of linkage has been used to map the location of genes onto
chromosomes. Prior to the identification of specific disease-causing mutations,
it could also be used in families for genetic testing. The use of linkage requires
that the:

■ family is sufficiently informative, i.e. there are enough affected and
unaffected members from whom samples can be obtained
■ gene of interest has been mapped to a specific chromosomal location
■ allele that is linked to the gene is sufficiently variable (or polymorphic)
for the inheritance to be determined.

The allele linked to the gene is called a genetic marker. Linkage techniques
using a variety of polymorphic genetic markers have been used to map the
human genome (*Figure 4.25*). Occasionally, the technique known as **Southern
blotting** is still used to perform linkage-based genetic testing in families
(described in *Appendix 3*).

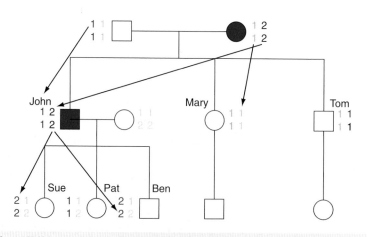

Figure 4.25. Linkage study (pedigree with haplotypes) showing inheritance from parent to child.

There are a number of different techniques for detecting mutations in genes, such as sequencing, protein truncation testing, mismatch cleavage, and heteroduplex gel mobility. If you are interested in more detailed information, see the texts listed in *Further resources* at the end of the chapter. Many DNA tests are complex and the laboratory may need to work with samples from a particular family for some months before a test is ordered for prenatal diagnosis or predictive testing.

4.8 Polygenic inheritance

If a characteristic is controlled by a single gene, a change in that gene will produce a distinct phenotype (a specific group of features or abnormalities). For some Mendelian traits, such as blood groups, there is more than one dominant allele but there are still several distinct phenotypes. In that case, the genotype (variations in several relevant genes) may still make a large contribution to the phenotype. However, for many human characteristics such as height, intelligence or skin colour, there is continuous variation usually following a normal distribution curve. Although there may be exceptional single alleles that cause extremes of variation, for example, single genes leading to learning disability or extreme short stature, the trait is usually controlled by more than one gene and environmental action is also important. For example, children tend to be about as tall as their parents, but a starved child would not be as tall as their well-nourished brothers and sisters. These continuous traits are said to be **polygenic** or **multifactorial** and are under the control of many genetic loci in interaction with the environment.

There are other traits which do not vary continuously but where the control of the trait is due to many genes, as well as environmental effects. The concept of a threshold effect is used to explain this. A trait such as a neural tube defect (spina bifida or **anencephaly**) is either present or absent. There are hypothesized genetic factors and known environmental factors that contribute to the risk. A combination of genotype, environment and other chance factors push some conceptions over the threshold from a fetus without a neural tube defect to one with. Diabetes and cancer are human diseases where there are known alleles that contribute to risk, but again there has to be a sufficient combination of risk factors to reach the threshold for disease.

4.9 Mitochondrial inheritance

This chapter has been concerned with the DNA within the nucleus of the cell. Within the cytoplasm of the cell (*Figure 4.26*) the mitochondria contain their own separate DNA. The **mitochondrial** genome is circular and contains much less DNA than the nuclear genome. Some of the proteins in mitochondria are under the control of the mitochondrial genome, but many are under the control of the nuclear genome. The unusual feature about mitochondria is that they are inherited from the mother not the father. A

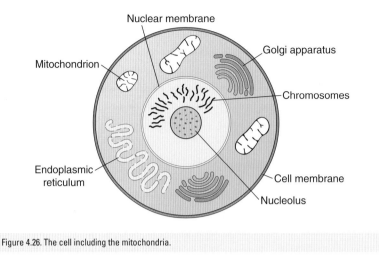

Figure 4.26. The cell including the mitochondria.

woman will pass on her mitochondria to her sons and daughters; her daughters will pass on their mitochondria, but her sons will not. This is because the oocyte contains mitochondria within its cytoplasm. The sperm passes on its nuclear DNA to the embryo but not its cytoplasmic DNA, because the mitochondria are in the tail of the sperm, which does not contribute to the fertilized ovum. Certain inherited human disorders show maternal inheritance and have been shown to be due to mitochondrial mutations. The mitochondrial gene sequence has been established. Mitochondrial DNA sequences and mutations have also been used to examine evolution and population movements as they provide an unbroken maternal link to our ancestors.

4.10 The Human Genome Project and beyond

The Human Genome Project was a unique international collaboration to determine the entire nucleotide sequence of the human genome. It originally arose because of the need to develop new mutation detection methods[23, 24]. The final product was a map which provides a guide for further research into the control of gene regulation, expression and function. Single gene disorders, which will theoretically be the easiest target for the development of novel therapies, are rare. Most common disorders are multifactorial, therefore caution should be exercised in predicting how soon important medical advances will be realized. However, with the sequencing of the human genome, the map and the tools are in place to embark on the research.

Many research findings are now being reported based on results from large scale projects looking at genetic variation between individuals. The findings from these studies show associations between genetic variants and common diseases, but there are concerns about how these findings are interpreted and used[25]. This is covered in more detail in *Chapter 5*.

4.11 **Treatment of genetic disease**

Developments in basic research have led to greater understanding of the biological mechanisms of some inherited diseases. This understanding is starting to lead to treatment, sometimes using existing drugs. Greater understanding of the specific mutations in some diseases is also starting to lead to the development of treatments which will either 'read through' the mutation, restoring gene function, or activate other related genes, which may partially restore function. This research has not yet translated into routine clinical practice, but it is very encouraging and some approaches are being tried in patients.

4.11.1 *Losartan and Marfan syndrome*

Marfan syndrome is a disorder of connective tissue in which some patients have progressive dilation of the aortic root which can be life threatening. In 1991 the gene was identified and mutations in the gene coding for a protein called fibrillin, a scaffolding protein, were found to be responsible. A series of findings from basic scientific research established that excess levels of a growth factor (TGF-β) interacted with fibrillin and led to reduced fibrillin. After a series of experiments using mouse models of Marfan syndrome, it was established that blocking TGF-β could stop the dilation of the aortic root. A drug already in existence and used for treating high blood pressure, Losartan, was known to block TGF-β and a trial in patients has started[26]. Preliminary results are encouraging.

Another hope for treatment of genetic disorders that generates much interest is stem cell therapy. Stem cells differ from other kinds of cells in the body. All stem cells have three main properties: they are capable of dividing and renewing themselves for long periods, they are unspecialized, but they can give rise to specialized cell types. However, there are still many obstacles to the wide-scale use of stem cells to produce functioning cells that could replace damaged cells, for example, in muscular dystrophy. These include how to make the cells proliferate and differentiate to generate sufficient quantities of tissue that can survive in the recipient, function appropriately, and cause no harm.

4.11.2 *Gene therapy*

While much is hoped in terms of gene therapy, at present such treatment is still in the realms of research rather than clinical service. The aim of gene therapy is to introduce a functioning copy of a gene into the body of the patient, so that it is able to function and repair the damage done by a faulty copy of the gene. Even where making a normal copy of the gene is possible, transporting it into the appropriate cells is more difficult. Some research involves inserting the gene into a virus, to enable it to be passed into cells. For example, gene therapy for cystic fibrosis involves introducing a normal copy of the gene into the tissues of the lung via a nebulizer. The therapy needs to be repeated at intervals and is not a lasting solution or cure. However, as techniques improve, so might this situation. Effective gene therapy is still many years away for most patients affected with a genetic disease. Other applications of gene therapy may provide treatments for cancer and infection.

4.12 Conclusion

The following chapters will illustrate the application of these genetic technologies to the real life situations affecting families. It is essential that healthcare professionals are able to understand the implications of these technologies for the families with which they are in contact. Only with this understanding will they be able to interpret both the limitations and the possibilities of these scientific advances.

Test yourself

Q1. Can you think of a possible genetic explanation for the higher incidence of trisomy in children of women who are over the age of 40 years, when compared with the offspring of younger mothers?

Q2. Describe the change to the normal human chromosome pattern designated by the following:

a)   47,XXY
b)   47,XY,+13
c)   47,XY,+21
d)   45,XX,der(13;14)(p11;q11)

Q3. How would the following be described in a cytogenetic report, using ISCN nomenclature?

a)   A normal female chromosome arrangement.
b)   A chromosome arrangement indicative of Edwards syndrome.
c)   A chromosome arrangement indicative of Turner syndrome.

Q4. A neonate is diagnosed as having a sub-microscopic microdeletion of chromosome 22q11.

a)   Name the laboratory tests that may have been done to identify the microdeletion.
b)   The parents plan to have another child and ask you about the risks of recurrence; how will you go about providing them with accurate information?

Q5. Why is only a very small sample of DNA required for a molecular test using PCR?

Further resources

www.geneticseducation.nhs.uk/learning/index.asp?id=122 – National Genetics Education and Development Centre. *Resources on basic science and inheritance patterns.*

www.ncbi.nlm.nih.gov/About/primer/genetics_molecular.html – NIH Science primer 'Molecular genetics, piecing it together'. *Helpful resource on basic structure of DNA and laboratory testing techniques.*

www.pathology.washington.edu/galleries/Cytogallery/ main.php?file=human%20karyotypes – Cytogenetics Gallery, Department of Pathology, University of Washington, Seattle. *Excellent resources on chromosomes and cytogenetics.*

Gardner A, Howell RT, Davies T (2009) *Human Genetics,* 2nd Edition. Oxford: Scion Publishing Ltd. *A very helpful basic book for those who require clear simple explanations of the genetics and laboratory techniques.*

Read AP, Donnai D (2007) *New Clinical Genetics.* Oxford: Scion Publishing Ltd. *Case-based approach which gives more depth of knowledge, particularly for genetic specialists.*

Strachan T, Read AP (2003) *Human Molecular Genetics,* 3rd Edition. London: Garland Science. *Very detailed account of principles of human genetics.*

Turnpenny P, Ellard S (2008) *Emery's Elements of Medical Genetics* 13th Edition. Edinburgh: Elsevier Churchill Livingstone. *Excellent overview of medical genetics.*

5 Public health genomics

5.1 Introduction

In the last few years there has been an increasing focus on how to put the very exciting discoveries from genetic research to use in healthcare. Research has produced potential new ways of predicting risk, of diagnosis, and possibly disease prevention and treatment. The complex relationship between genes and environment and their role in the development of chronic conditions such as cardiovascular disease, cancer and diabetes is slowly being understood. These conditions have a high impact on overall population health. Public health practice includes activities such as needs assessment, health promotion, disease prevention programs, and evaluation and routine collection of health data for monitoring and auditing. Traditionally it has taken account of the complexity of environmental factors and also the wider ethical, legal and social concerns in framing responses to health needs. The integration of genetics into this has become the area of concern of public health genomics. An international definition of public health genomics is:

> *"The responsible and effective translation of genome-based knowledge for the benefit of population health."* Bellagio Workshop, April 2005[27]

The aim of public health genomics is to combine the scientific knowledge from basic research with knowledge from public health and social sciences, ethics, and humanities to develop programs and policies to improve health (*Figure 5.1*). This integrated knowledge contributes to

- service development
- education and training
- informing public policy
- communication and stakeholder engagement

Examples of where public health genomics could contribute include screening programs for genetic diseases, development and monitoring of genetic services, registers for the collection of information on congenital anomalies, or genotype–phenotype data.

Much of the research in genetics to date has been in discovering disease-causing genes or genetic variation that is associated with disease. This has led to many more tests for diagnosis and prediction being made available. There is also of course the often raised promise of personalized medicine and the

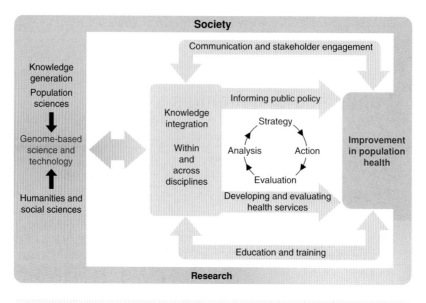

Figure 5.1. Processes involved in Public Health Genomics. Reproduced with permission from the PHGF.

developing market in tests for susceptibility, some of which are sold directly to the consumer. One particular area of concern is the evaluation of genetic tests. It should be pointed out that developments in systems and methods for evaluating genetic tests are also relevant to all tests used to diagnose, treat or predict disease.

5.2 Evaluation of genetic tests

When considering whether or not to use a test it is important to understand that a test is more than just the laboratory analysis. It is the process of using the results of the laboratory analysis for a particular disease, for a particular purpose, in a particular population. One of the early frameworks that was developed as a way of evaluating genetic tests was the ACCE framework – this separated out the components of the test into analytical validity, clinical validity, clinical utility, and ethical, legal and social aspects.

Analytic validity. Does it measure what it says it measures?

Clinical validity (scientific validity, clinical outcome). Does what it measures accurately predict a clinical endpoint?

Clinical utility. Is it worth doing? Does it make a difference?

Ethical, legal, social aspects[28]. Is it acceptable from the legal, ethical and social perspectives within that particular setting and population?

In deciding whether or not to use a test it is important to be able to evaluate:

- the assay
- the clinical validity, including clinical test performance
- the clinical utility, including test purpose and feasibility of test delivery[29]

For example, genetic analysis may be able to detect a particular change in DNA sequence which is found in 90% of people with a BMI greater than 30. The DNA analysis is very accurate and will always detect this change, if it is present. It might be thought that this would be a very useful thing to know. However, this change is also found in 60% of people with a BMI less than 30. It is therefore absolutely no use at all in predicting whether someone will become obese or not. Even if it had a greater clinical utility, there would still be legitimate concern if it was suggested that using the test for prenatal diagnosis would be a reasonable way to reduce the effects of the impact of obesity on overall population health. The above hypothetical example illustrates that even if an assay is very accurate it still may be no use as a test, either because it does not accurately predict the disease of interest, or because its use is unacceptable.

CASE EXAMPLE   **ANNE**

Anne came to the genetic clinic because her husband had recently died from liver cancer. Two months before his death he had been told that he had hereditary hemochromatosis. He had been complaining of tiredness and loss of energy for some time, although it was not until he was being investigated for liver disease that it was discovered that he had excess iron in his liver. He had a number of investigations including a genetic test for the hemochromatosis gene – this showed that he was homozygous for the common change in the gene. He was devastated to find that if he had been diagnosed earlier, and treated (simply by removing blood to remove the excess iron), then his liver might not have been so damaged and he might not have developed cancer. Anne has two children in their late teens and wanted to know the risk for them. The genetic counselor explained that the genetic change was very common, about 1 in 10 people from Northern Europe carried it. Her two sons would only be at risk if Anne carried the gene change and so she could be tested or, alternatively, her sons could be tested as they were old enough to give consent. Anne talked a lot in the session about how unfair it was that her husband was diagnosed late, and that she thought everyone should be tested for the genetic change to stop any other family going through what they had gone through. The genetic counselor empathized with Anne and decided that she would talk with the genetic service about seeing if population screening for the gene would be possible. When she had done some more reading, however, she realized that it was very complicated. Although it was true that hemochromatosis was often diagnosed quite late and that the genetic test was very useful in diagnosing someone who already had evidence of high iron levels in their blood, there was debate as to whether the genetic test was useful in detecting people from the general population. The problem was that the gene change was very common and only a very small proportion of people with the gene change would develop iron overload. As the genetic service manager pointed out, you could test 10,000 people, detect 30 people who had two copies of the genetic change, and perhaps prevent disease in two of them at the most. It would be valuable for those two people, but at what cost to the 28 who would be told they had a genetic risk and would have to have their iron levels regularly monitored, let alone the actual cost of testing the 10,000 who were negative. The genetic counselor decided she would work with Anne and the patient support group to publicize information about hemochromatosis, with the aim of raising awareness of it as a possible diagnosis and also giving information about where the tests could be carried out.

In this section we have talked about frameworks that are used to decide which tests to provide within healthcare settings. For example, the UK Genetic Testing Network (UKGTN) uses a similar framework to advise the National Health Service about which tests should be provided[30]. More recently there has been an expansion of companies offering genetic tests directly to the consumer without necessarily involving a medical practitioner. This has led to much commentary in the scientific and general press.

5.3 Direct to consumer genetic testing

Companies and private health screening services have translated the findings from genome-wide association studies into tests which claim to offer health-related information or lifestyle choice. Concerns have been raised as to the scientific and clinical validity of the tests, their usefulness, and the appropriate response from regulators and commentators[31]. A variety of international and national bodies have produced working papers and documents in this rapidly changing area[32]. There is a broad agreement on the need for:

- standards when assessing the evidence for the clinical validity of the tests
- transparent evidence
- appropriate provision of information for the consumer
- quality standards to use to monitor the test providers and the information they produce
- standards for appropriate advice and advertising

It will be interesting to see how this market develops over the years and what the actual demand is for people to have personalized information relating to their future health.

5.4 Implications for practice

The aim of public health genomics is the responsible translation of advances in genetic science into individual and population health benefit. This requires the integration of knowledge from many different disciplines and specialties. The healthcare practitioner needs to be aware of these developments and also be willing to participate in decisions about how they are to be implemented, both with their individual patient and at the level of provision of services.

Test yourself

Q1. Name four of the criteria used to evaluate genetic tests before they are offered to the population.

Further resources

www.cdc.gov/genomics/ – The National Office of Public Health Genomics (NOPHG). *This is part of the CDC in the USA.*

www.humgen.umontreal.ca – HumGen International Database. *Database on the legal, ethical and social aspects of human genetics, developed as a collaboration between academia, government and industry by the Centre de Recherche en Droit Public at the University of Montreal.*

www.phgfoundation.org/ – PHG Foundation (Foundation for Genomics and Population Health). *The PHG Foundation is an independent international charity working to achieve the responsible and evidence-based application of biomedical science for health. They undertake and fund research, policy analysis, education, and service development projects.*

Khoury M, Little J, Burke W (2004) *Human Genome Epidemiology*. Oxford: Oxford University Press.

Stewart A, Brice P, Burton H, Pharoah P, Sanderson S, Zimmern R (2007) *Genetics, Health Care and Public Policy: An Introduction to Public Health Genetics*. Cambridge: Cambridge University Press.

6 Before conception

6.1 Introduction

The aim of pre-conceptual care is to identify situations where the parents (particularly the mother) or the fetus may be at an additional health risk during pregnancy, and to take steps to minimize that risk before conception occurs, if possible. In some cases, the risk cannot be altered but the parents have the opportunity to absorb the information relating to their situation and to think about potential options available to them.

Pre-conceptual care and counseling for couples who are planning a family can be beneficial for several reasons:
- it enables high-risk situations to be identified prior to pregnancy occurring; this usually gives the couple more possible options for action
- it enables the couple to think about difficult decisions before they have an emotional investment in a current pregnancy
- it enables the healthcare team to be prepared for additional care or possible testing during a pregnancy

Whilst dedicated 'pre-conceptual clinics' are not yet widely used by couples planning a pregnancy, there are a great number of opportunities that exist for healthcare professionals to offer information and advice that might alter the outcome of a future pregnancy. Professionals who may routinely encounter situations where pre-conceptual advice may be offered include:
- nurses or doctors working in family planning clinics, who will meet women who are currently using contraception but may wish to start a pregnancy within the next few years
- health visitors, who are caring for families after the birth of one child and who may wish to increase their family
- midwives, following the birth of a baby
- general practitioners, in the course of providing routine healthcare for the family
- fertility clinic doctors and nurses, as couples seeking advice will be hoping to achieve a pregnancy
- nurses working in gynecology or genito-urinary clinics
- practice nurses, for example, when undertaking cervical smear tests
- school nurses, when providing health education

Obviously, in each of these situations the relevance and opportunity to offer pre-conceptual counseling will vary, but an awareness of the possibility of offering information prior to pregnancy should not be overlooked. General health education that may improve the outcome for the fetus and mother can be offered by any relevant health professional. This should include:

- general information about a healthy diet
- promotion of regular exercise
- advice on restriction of alcohol use in pregnancy and advice on cessation of cigarette smoking prior to conception, because of the proven adverse effects on fetal growth
- information about the use of medication or dietary supplements (including vitamins) during pregnancy; many women will, for example, be unaware of the potential for toxicity from an overdose of fat-soluble vitamins
- a review of prescribed medication being used by the mother to assess its safety in pregnancy
- advice on the use of folic acid prior to conception (discussed further later in this chapter)
- avoiding exposure to infection that may adversely affect the fetus, such as listeria, CMV and toxoplasmosis

In addition to this general advice, a simple enquiry about whether either prospective parent has a family history of any genetic condition can enable specific concerns to be addressed before a pregnancy. In cases where the health professional is unsure of the relevance of a family history, the staff of genetic services are generally happy to discuss the situation informally and advise whether referral to genetic services is warranted.

CASE EXAMPLE **CYPROS FAMILY**

George and Anna are newly-married. They both come from families who originated in Cyprus.

George and Anna knew nothing about thalassemia when they married, but when they were on holiday in Cyprus (a gift from Anna's father), they met Anna's distant relations. One of Anna's cousins, a young man called Michael, has beta thalassemia, and Michael's mother told them the disease was inherited.

Back home in the UK, Anna and George ask about thalassemia when they next go to the family planning clinic for Anna's oral contraceptive pill. The nurse offers to refer them to the sickle cell and thalassemia center. The thalassemia counselor explains the condition to them, and offers them carrier testing. They both agree that they would rather know now if their future children are at risk, and so they have blood taken. Deep down, George does not believe there is any cause for concern, as there is 'nothing like that in my family'. Anna has the test 'just to give me peace of mind'.

Four weeks later George and Anna return to the thalassemia center and are told that they are both carriers of beta thalassemia. They are stunned, and hardly take in what they are being told. The counselor arranges to see them again a month later.

At the next meeting, Anna is able to think about the options, but George is still not really ready. They decide that they will delay having a family for some time, and will talk to the counselor before Anna comes off the pill. Two years later, Anna and George return to the clinic. After further discussion about treatment of thalassemia, they decide to have a baby, without any form of prenatal testing. The baby is tested at birth for thalassemia. She is unaffected. In their second pregnancy they opt for a test, stating that they have realised since becoming parents how hard it would be to have a child who constantly needed additional care. They also don't feel they should 'try our luck twice'. The second child is also unaffected.

6.2 Maternal age

Maternal age can have an influence on the health of both the mother and the fetus. The older mother may be more prone to complications because of underlying medical conditions. For example, a mother in her 40s will be more likely to be affected by hypertension, varicose veins or stress incontinence than a woman in her 20s.

From the fetal perspective, chromosomal abnormalities are much more likely to occur in the fetus of an older mother. The risk of all chromosome abnormalities increases with maternal age, because the chance of a non-disjunction event increases with the age of the oocytes (egg-producing cells).

Amniocentesis used to be offered to women above a certain age. This was usually 35–37 years, but did vary according to local policy. With the advent of ultrasound scanning and maternal serum screening, this has altered as screening has been made available to pregnant women of all ages. However, before starting a pregnancy, couples who seek pre-conceptual counseling should be aware of the increased risks to the fetus of a chromosomal abnormality due to maternal age effect.

6.3 Neural tube defects and the role of folic acid in lowering the risk

The neural tube includes the brain and the spinal cord. This develops early in fetal life, and interruption to closure of the tube causes both spina bifida and anencephaly. Closure of the neural tube begins in the area of the cervical spine, with the spinal column forming distally in the direction to the coccyx, while the cranium closes over the brain. Failure of this process results in a neural tube defect (NTD). While the appearance and effects of spina bifida and anencephaly differ, they are considered to be different manifestations of the same type of malformation, and are grouped under the term neural tube defect.

In the absence of other abnormalities in the fetus, NTDs are not inherited as a Mendelian disorder, in that they do not follow one of the known patterns of inheritance. However, empirical data show that couples who have one child with a NTD are at greater risk of having a second child with a NTD than other couples in the general population. Following the diagnosis of one child with a NTD, the risk of NTD in each subsequent pregnancy for that couple is about 4%. However, the risk can be lowered dramatically (to about 1%) by maternal folic acid supplements.

In 1991, a study of the effect of maternal supplements of folic acid on the rate of NTDs in their offspring was reported[33]. The randomized control trial had to be abandoned before the end of the study as it became very clear that folic acid was having an effect in reducing the number of children born with spina bifida. It was therefore unethical to continue to place women in the control group, as this was knowingly exposing the fetus of each of those women to greater risk.

Since that time, it has been recommended that women who may become pregnant take folic acid daily for at least 2 months before conception, and for the first 12 weeks of pregnancy. The dose for women whose risk of having a child with a NTD is considered to be at the population level is about 0.4 mg daily, but women whose children appear to be at higher risk are advised to take 4–5 mg per day.

Observational studies in populations before and after fortification of food with folic acid (normally cereal products) demonstrate a reduction of up to 50% in the incidence of NTDs. The greatest reduction occurs in areas of highest prevalence[34]. However, whilst dietary advice is important, increasing the levels of folic acid in the maternal diet is not considered sufficient, as the rate of NTD does not appear to vary significantly with maternal diet. It may be that some women do not absorb folic acid from the diet as well as others.

Folic acid supplements are advised pre-conceptually because it takes some weeks to raise the maternal levels, and because the neural tube has already started to form before the mother is aware of her pregnancy. This of course means that some women will be taking folic acid for many months, even years, before conception occurs. As a B-group vitamin, excess folic acid is excreted in the urine, and toxic levels do not therefore occur in the mother.

If a woman who has not been taking folic acid supplements becomes pregnant, she should start taking the supplements and continue until she is 12 weeks pregnant, although disruption to the normal formation of the neural tube may already have occurred. Folic acid tablets in the 0.4 mg dose are often available in the UK and other countries 'over the pharmacy counter', but higher dose tablets may only be provided on prescription.

The mechanism by which folic acid has its effect on the neural tube is not clear and genetic factors are important. There is much research in this area but as yet there is little conclusive evidence of which particular genes have a major effect. Other environmental risk factors that are associated with an increased risk of NTDs include maternal diabetes and maternal **teratogens** such as anti-epileptic medication. Prospective mothers who have had a previous child with a NTD, or who are on anti-epileptic medication or are diabetic, should be prescribed the higher dose because of their higher risk of having a child with a NTD.

> ## KEY PRACTICE POINT
>
> Women who may become pregnant should be advised to take folic acid for at least 2 months before conception and for the first 12 weeks of pregnancy.

6.4 Genetic conditions affecting the mother

6.4.1 Skeletal dysplasia

There are a large number of different types of skeletal dysplasia. This is a term used to describe a number of conditions in which the skeleton forms in an unusual way, causing bony deformity. The genetic code for the formation of the skeleton is faulty. A child may be at risk of skeletal dysplasia if either parent is affected, but if the mother is affected then pre-conceptual care is useful as the condition of the pelvis and spine can be assessed prior to pregnancy. The bony deformity may affect the lie of the fetus in the third trimester, and may make passage of the fetus through the birth canal difficult in labour. As the fetus should not be exposed to X-rays, examination and investigation of the mother prior to pregnancy is important. The management of the pregnancy and delivery can then be planned. Most skeletal dysplasias are due to a genetic cause. There may be very serious potential risks for the baby if both parents have a skeletal dysplasia and, in addition to considering the physical health of the mother, the healthcare professional should seek expert advice as to the risks to the baby.

6.4.2 Connective tissue disorders

The management of pregnancy in women with a connective tissue disorder (such as Ehlers–Danlos syndrome and Marfan syndrome) is discussed more fully in *Chapter 7*. There are two main issues concerned with the management of pregnancy, and it is useful to have discussed these before conception. First, the woman should have a baseline cardiac assessment if the condition is one in which cardiac complications can occur. Secondly, tissue friability should be assessed, because stretching of the uterine tissue in pregnancy may lead to uterine rupture, and if this is a significant risk the couple should be aware of this before pregnancy occurs.

6.4.3 Maternal diabetes

Maternal diabetes is known to affect the growth and development of the fetus, and in poorly controlled diabetic mothers there is an increase in the rate of spontaneous abortions. Intra-uterine growth retardation occurs more frequently in the babies of diabetic mothers, but the exact mechanism for this slowing of growth is not yet known. However, rather than being a direct effect of abnormal glucose levels, it is more likely to be due to a complex interaction between glucose levels, ketone bodies and decreased availability of insulin. Macrosomia of the fetus may also occur, increasing the risk of complications during labor and delivery.

Congenital malformations occur significantly more frequently occur in infants of diabetic mothers; in fact the risk is between 2 and 4 times the population risk. The teratogenic effects seem to occur very early in the pregnancy (up to the seventh week). For this reason pre-conceptual counseling of diabetic mothers is helpful, since the most critical period often occurs before the mother is aware of the pregnancy. Strict control of blood glucose levels has been shown to decrease the rate of congenital malformations. In a regime designed to eliminate *hyper*glycemia, *hypo*glycemia may sometimes occur, but this is not thought to be detrimental to the fetus, and is preferable to hyperglycemia[35]. They should also be encouraged to take high dose folic acid to reduce the risk of NTD.

6.4.4 Epilepsy

Epilepsy is a condition which is thought to be multi-factorial, and the offspring of a person with epilepsy has a greater chance than others in the general population of developing the condition. However, it is not inherited as a single gene disorder. If a mother has epilepsy, there is a danger of fetal hypoxia during a fit, and therefore the aim of treatment must be to avoid seizures during the pregnancy. The prospective mother should be advised to try and stabilize the epilepsy before conception to reduce the possibility of fits.

Of course, the use of drug therapy is not without additional risk to the fetus, as many anti-convulsants are known to cause serious congenital abnormalities. The evidence appears to indicate that use of more than one drug to control the epilepsy increases the risk to the fetus. The aim therefore is to stabilize the mother prior to pregnancy, if possible on the drug that is least harmful to the fetus. Before pregnancy, a woman with epilepsy should therefore always be referred to a physician experienced in the care of patients with epilepsy who can address this matter. Women who are taking anti-convulsants are in the group considered to be at increased risk of having a child with a NTD and should therefore be prescribed high dose folic acid (5 mg daily), to be taken pre-conceptually for at least two months and for the first three months of pregnancy.

> **CASE EXAMPLE   JODI**
>
> Jodi is a 27-year-old woman who is married to Steven. They have been together from their teens and plan to start a family. Jodi has been epileptic since the age of 7 years, and is on carbamezipine. Controlling her epilepsy has been very difficult but this drug seems to be effective.
>
> Jodi asks her family doctor about the risks of her epilepsy being passed on to her children, and he refers her to the genetic counselor in the local genetics service. Jodi confides that she is really worried about her child being disabled but the counselor tells her that the risk of her children having epilepsy is low. The counselor discusses the risks of congenital abnormalities due to the anti-convulsants. These include clefting, spina bifida and learning difficulties. Jodi is referred back to her physician for review of her medication, but alteration to her drug therapy is not possible as most other anti-convulsants have been tried in her case.
>
> Jodi and Steven decide to go ahead and Jodi becomes pregnant several months later. A detailed scan is ordered at 18 weeks gestation, and the fetus is found to have a NTD. Steven and Jodi have already decided that they cannot raise a child with physical disabilities, and terminate the pregnancy.

6.5 Maternal drug therapy

It is not possible to list all the drugs with potentially harmful effects on the fetus. Each case needs to be treated individually, and an assessment made of the benefits to the mother and fetus, as opposed to the possible adverse effects. Obviously any drug therapy that is not strictly necessary to maintain the health of the mother should be avoided in pregnancy. Details of the potential effects of drugs and possible alternative drugs can be obtained through a pharmacist. In some situations, alternative therapies such as aromatherapy or acupressure may be helpful.

6.6 Consanguinity

Pre-conceptual advice may be sought by couples who are related biologically (consanguineous couples). There appears to be a great deal of traditional superstition attached to cousin marriage in some communities, making the couple apprehensive about the genetic advice they may receive. In other ethnic groups, cousin marriage is the norm. In fact, consanguineous couples are only slightly more likely to have a child with a genetic condition than other unrelated couples. They are at increased risk of having a child with a recessive condition, as both parents could carry the same faulty gene, inherited from the common grandparent or great grandparent (*Figure 6.1*). All couples have a 2–3% chance of having a child with a serious health concern, and couples who are first cousins have a risk of about 5%. The children of second cousins (or

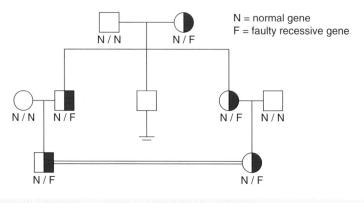

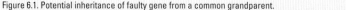

Figure 6.1. Potential inheritance of faulty gene from a common grandparent.

those who are more distantly related) will be at less risk of a recessive condition. If there is any evidence of a recessive genetic condition in the family, carrier testing for both partners may be indicated.

In some states in the United States, first cousin marriage is illegal. In the United Kingdom there is no legal barrier to marrying a cousin, but marriage between closer relatives such as between siblings, parent/child, grandparent/grandchild, uncle/niece or aunt/nephew is not permitted

6.7 Preparing for prenatal diagnosis

One important aspect of pre-conceptual care relates to families where there is a known genetic risk. Although a great number of genetic conditions occur sporadically, in many cases there is a family history of a condition. If a couple present with a history of a disorder, whether this has occurred in a previous child of theirs or in members of their families, they should be referred to genetic services for assessment and information.

Where the couple would wish to have prenatal diagnostic testing on the fetus, preparatory work needs to be undertaken. The laboratory will often require samples from family members prior to the testing, to enable the pattern of genetic markers in the family to be ascertained, or to enable the relevant gene mutation to be identified. It is not uncommon for this work to take several months. It is only after this preliminary work is done that the family can be offered the opportunity to have prenatal diagnosis with certainty. Of equal or even greater importance is the preparatory emotional work and decision-making that should preferably be undertaken by the couple before the pregnancy. The genetics team will discuss the options with the family, and support them in making the decisions about testing that are best for them in their unique circumstances. If the couple want to consider prenatal diagnosis, they should be advised to contact their midwife or doctor as soon as the pregnancy is confirmed, so that arrangements for early scanning (to assess gestation accurately) and testing can be made. When testing for rare disorders, the laboratory needs to be aware that a test is planned so that staff and materials can be made ready.

KEY PRACTICE POINT

Any couple that is concerned about a genetic risk to their future children should be referred to the genetic service **before** pregnancy whenever possible so that preparations can be made for prenatal diagnostic tests, and so the couple can discuss their options.

CASE EXAMPLE **SUZANNE AND HELEN**

Suzanne and Helen are sisters. When Helen became pregnant for the first time, her midwife asked her about a family history of any genetic condition, and Helen told her that her younger brother had muscular dystrophy. The midwife referred her for genetic counseling.

Helen was found to be a carrier of Duchenne muscular dystrophy, an **X-linked** genetic condition that causes death in the late teens. Helen and her husband decided to have a prenatal test, and the male fetus was found to have inherited the condition. Helen and her husband reluctantly decided to terminate the pregnancy. This was very difficult as they had been overjoyed at the confirmation of the pregnancy, with no real knowledge about the risk to the baby. Helen's sister Suzanne asked to see the genetic nurse. She had been attending an infertility clinic for 3 years and was currently receiving clomiphene therapy to help her conceive. She had no idea she might be a carrier of the condition that affected her brother. She was also found to be a carrier of Duchenne muscular dystrophy. She discontinued therapy, as clomiphene greatly increases the risk of multiple pregnancy and she could not face the thought of terminating several babies or of selective feticide. Suzanne felt angry that the risk of muscular dystrophy had never been discussed with her prior to her infertility treatment.

6.8 Pre-implantation genetic diagnosis

Pre-implantation genetic diagnosis (PGD) is a relatively new technique used to avoid passing on an inherited disease. It is only offered in a few specialist centers but it is an option for couples who, for whatever reason, find prenatal diagnosis with termination of affected pregnancies unacceptable. PGD is a technology which allows genetic testing of an embryo prior to implantation. It is used in conjunction with IVF and allows only those embryos diagnosed as being free of a specific genetic disorder to be transferred into a woman for pregnancy. A couple who know they are at risk of having a baby with an inherited condition opt to have IVF treatment even though they are probably fertile. When the embryos are about 3 days old they are tested for the specific inherited condition and only those without the gene are replaced[36].

In the US, PGD is permitted but medical care is usually governed by State, rather than Federal, government policies, and the basis of offering this type of treatment may therefore vary from state to state. However, PGD is offered by reproductive medicine clinics in many states for a wide range of conditions.

Fertility treatment in the UK is licensed by the Human Fertilisation and Embryology Authority (HFEA). The HFEA regulates and oversees the use of gametes and embryos in fertility treatment and research. The HFEA also issues licenses on a condition by condition basis for PGD. In general PGD is used for those couples that wish to avoid having a child with a known genetic problem. There have also been requests for the technology to be used to select embryos that will be a tissue match and donor for an existing child who has a serious life threatening disease – to produce so called 'saviour siblings'. In 2002 the HFEA gave a license for embryo selection in a case where the technology was used to both screen for the genetic condition and to ensure a good match for the sick sibling. In 2004 it gave permission for the procedure to be used for embryo selection with the sole purpose of finding a match for a sibling. This clearly is a very contentious issue and, along with more general concerns about 'designer babies', has provoked much debate. Some of the concerns relate to the morality of creating a child purely as a source of donated material for an existing child. The counter argument is that the child would be wanted and cared for in its own right and would not be created solely as a donor of tissue. In the UK at the time of writing the Act of Parliament governing the HFEA is under review and these issues are being hotly debated[37].

6.9 Issues of fertility

There are a number of genetic conditions which are known to cause sub-fertility or infertility. These include conditions related to imbalance of the sex chromosomes such as Turner syndrome in the female (45,X) and Klinefelter syndrome in the male (47,XXY). Female carriers of fragile X may experience premature ovarian failure, and males with cystic fibrosis may have oligospermia or complete absence of the vas deferens. New reproductive technologies may be able to assist these clients to have a child, although in many cases this is still not possible. It is always worthwhile offering such couples a referral to an **assisted reproduction** unit for assessment, whilst not raising inappropriate expectations.

The use of assisted reproduction techniques has raised new issues for infertile men, as it is now thought that male infertility is often the result of a gene mutation on the Y chromosome. Previously men who carried this mutation would not have had the chance of passing it on to their offspring, but with the new methods they are able to have children and thus produce sons who are similarly infertile.

If a mother presents having already had several miscarriages, a balanced chromosome translocation in one of the parents should be suspected (see *Chapter 4*). Chromosome studies for both parents should be offered.

6.10 Adoption

There are two main aspects of adoption that require some consideration in relation to genetics. First, the rights of both the child and the prospective parents should be considered when a child with a genetic condition is offered for adoption. It is desirable that the parents be given full and appropriate information about the effects of the condition and the prognosis for the child, in order to make adequate provision for the care of that child. It is our experience that adoptive parents of a severely disabled child approach the child's condition differently to natural parents, perhaps because natural parents may feel an element of guilt, which is not present in adoptive parents.

Secondly, there are issues that may arise if a parent who is affected by or at risk of a genetic condition wishes to adopt a child. It is the responsibility of those arranging the adoption to make an assessment in the best interests of the child, and therefore these genetic factors may be taken into account. For example, if a prospective parent is at risk of a condition that might seriously affect their ability to parent, the adoption agency may not approve the adoption. This can be very difficult for couples who wish to avoid having a child at risk of the condition, and who then feel they are at a disadvantage in terms of the possibility of adoption as well.

6.11 Conclusion

This chapter has addressed the issues that might arise prior to conception, and has emphasized the need for pre-conceptual care in a variety of situations. There is much that can be done pre-conceptually to help a couple achieve a healthy pregnancy, and planning for prenatal genetic testing is much better done before the woman is pregnant. The next chapter will focus on the genetic issues of relevance during pregnancy.

Test yourself

Q1. A couple known to you through your daily practice tell you that they would like to have a baby. Both partners have a mild learning disability. What issues would you discuss with them, to maximize the chances of them having a healthy baby?

Q2. Through your own research, find out the recommendations for pre-conceptual folic acid supplementation in your own region. What would be the recommended dose for:

a) a woman with no history of neural tube defect
b) a women who has had a child with spina bifida

Further resources

http://depts.washington.edu/druginfo/Formulary/Pregnancy.pdf – FDA pregnancy categories and teratogens. *List of potential teratogens classified by US FDA.*

www.hfea.gov.uk/ – Human Fertilisation and Embryology Authority

www.library.nhs.uk/geneticconditions – National Library for Health (genetic conditions). *Web portal and resource with summaries of news and policy.*

www.phgfoundation.org – PHG Foundation

MRC Vitamin Study Research Group (1991) Prevention of neural tube defects: results of the MRC vitamin study. *Lancet,* **338**: 132–7. *Report of the original research on folic acid supplements, containing information on neural tube defect.*

7 Pregnancy and the perinatal period

7.1 Introduction

Genetic counseling is often inextricably linked in the minds of health professionals with reproduction. Whilst it is hoped that this book will help to illustrate that genetic issues are of relevance to people in all stages of life, it is clear that many families with concerns about a genetic condition will seek information during pregnancy and in the weeks after birth. A significant number of families will become aware of their genetic risk for the first time during that period, as a result of family history taking, antenatal screening, ultrasound scanning or congenital abnormalities diagnosed in a newborn. In this chapter, we will describe common situations where genetic conditions may become apparent, the types of tests available and some guidelines for good practice.

7.2 Care of the mother during pregnancy

During pregnancy, the midwife has a responsibility to ascertain whether the mother or fetus is at any particular risk of a genetic condition. When booking the mother for antenatal care, it is good practice to ask relevant questions in a systematic way to ascertain whether there may be an increased risk of a genetic condition in the family. The types of questions are included in the National Maternity Record (NMR) used by many midwives in the UK (see *Further resources*). An appropriate checklist can be used to facilitate taking a genetic history and can also provide guidelines for action by the midwife, should any concerns be raised. One such example was developed by the multi-disciplinary Joint Committee on Medical Genetics in the UK (*Figure 7.1*).

If the pregnant woman has a genetic condition, this may alter the management of the pregnancy. Due to improved healthcare, women with serious inherited conditions may now be sufficiently healthy to enable them to conceive and carry a pregnancy to term. These mothers should always be jointly managed by an obstetric team experienced in the care of women with high-risk pregnancies and a physician experienced in the care of patients with the particular condition. Some specific examples are discussed below.

Questions related to the mother's care:

Diabetes	No/Yes
Blood clotting problems (DVT, PE)	No/Yes
Stillbirth/multiple miscarriages	No/Yes

If considered significant, referral to a consultant obstetrician should be considered.

Questions related to a risk to the fetus:
Has anyone in either your own family or your partner's (the baby's father) family:

	Your family	Partner's family
A disease that runs in families?	Yes/No	Yes/No
Been seen by a geneticist or genetic counselor	Yes/No	Yes/No
Had learning difficulties (e.g. needed special help at school)	Yes/No	Yes/No
Had a baby with abnormalities present at birth	Yes/No	Yes/No
Had more than two stillbirths or miscarriages	Yes/No	Yes/No

If considered significant, referral to an obstetrician, fetal medicine or clinical genetics specialist should be considered:

Serum screening	Offered: Yes/No	Accepted: Yes/No (result)
Ultrasound scan	Offered: Yes/No	Accepted: Yes/No (result)

Sickle cell and/or thalassemia carrier screening offered/accepted

Figure 7.1. Checklist of genetic conditions to be used by the midwife when booking a woman for antenatal care.

7.2.1 Marfan syndrome

Marfan syndrome is a dominant condition that affects a number of different body systems. The genetic defect adversely affects the development of connective tissue, namely collagen. Due to extreme variability of expression of the gene mutation, the effects of the condition may vary greatly from person to person, even within the same family. Marfan syndrome causes tall stature, hypermobility of the joints, cardiovascular abnormalities (notably dilated aortic root and aortic aneurysm), and dislocated lenses. Due to the joint laxity and stature, serious back pain in pregnancy may become a problem. The mother with Marfan syndrome who has an existing cardiovascular abnormality should, of course, be under the care of a cardiologist, who should be made aware of the pregnancy. However, if Marfan syndrome is suspected or diagnosed, and the mother is not under the care of a cardiologist, then an urgent referral should be made for cardiac assessment. Sudden death from cardiovascular complications (such as dissection of the aorta) may occur during pregnancy or in the postnatal period in untreated cases[38].

7.2.2 Ehlers–Danlos syndrome

The term Ehlers–Danlos syndrome (EDS) refers to a group of disorders of connective tissue. Whilst hyperextensibility of skin, increased mobility of joints and tissue fragility are common features, the severity of the condition varies widely, with Type IV (vascular type) having the most serious implications for women in pregnancy[39]. In fact, for women know to have Type IV EDS, the mortality rate in any pregnancy is estimated to be 20%[40] and a termination of pregnancy may be offered to reduce the risk to the mother's life.

Women with EDS may be at higher risk of spontaneous abortion and stillbirth. It is thought that collagen in the chorionic membranes is affected by some forms of the condition, making premature rupture of membranes more likely. Due to the fragility of vessel walls, women with the condition (especially the vascular type) will also be at increased risk of hemorrhage antenatally and during labour. The joint laxity experienced by these women may result in dislocation of the symphysis pubis, whilst the frailty of other tissues makes varicose veins and abdominal herniae more common in this group of patients. Additional monitoring of the mother during labour is indicated because of the risk of uterine rupture. Early Cesarean section (as early as 32 weeks[39]) may be planned for women with Type IV EDS to reduce the chance of major vascular rupture during labour and delivery[40]. Wound dehiscence may occur after either Cesarean section or vaginal delivery, and the use of additional support such as tapes or non-absorbable sutures is advised to reduce the risk of this complication[41].

It is essential that any pregnant woman who has possible features or a family history of EDS is referred to an appropriate specialist for assessment and management of her condition during and after pregnancy.

7.2.3 Maternal phenylketonuria

Phenylketonuria (PKU) is a recessive condition, wherein the biochemical pathway involved in the metabolism of phenylalanine is disturbed, causing increased phenylalanine levels in the affected person. The accumulation of phenylalanine in the body results in mental retardation. However, the use of a low phenylalanine diet during infancy, childhood and adolescence will dramatically reduce the risk of mental retardation.

It has been shown that high maternal levels of phenylalanine during pregnancy have adverse effects on the fetus, causing microcephaly, mental retardation, dysmorphic features, and congenital heart disease. Whilst women with PKU who are planning a pregnancy can revert to the diet some months before conceiving, thus reducing serum phenylalanine levels, in an unplanned pregnancy the fetus would already be exposed to high phenylalanine levels before the pregnancy is diagnosed. To reduce the risk to their offspring, it is strongly advised that women are encouraged to remain on a low phenylalanine diet to maintain a serum phenylalanine level of 120–360 µmol/l, at least until they have completed their families[42,43].

7.2.4 Cystic fibrosis

Cystic fibrosis (CF) is the most common recessive condition occurring in many populations of white European origin. The gene mutation causes a disturbance of chloride, sodium and water ratios in specific body secretions, resulting primarily in respiratory infections, reduced lung function, and reduced pancreatic function. Improved management of CF has enabled some affected women to live into adulthood and maintain sufficiently good health to consider having a family.

Where the mother's lung function is normal, the CF does not appear to confer significantly higher risks to mother or fetus. However, where there is impaired function there is a greater risk of prematurity for the fetus, and therapeutic abortion may be considered to preserve the mother's health. Mothers with CF are prone to developing diabetes and this should be borne in mind when caring for such women. It is important that the mother should be under the care of a respiratory specialist for monitoring at least monthly during the pregnancy[44].

7.2.5 Hemoglobinopathy

Thalassemia major. In most centers caring for women with thalassemia, a protocol will be used for treatment with a series of blood transfusions. Iron chelation therapy (desferrioxamine) will also usually be administered to maintain stable serum ferritin levels. Cardiac problems, diabetes and hepatitis C may additionally complicate the pregnancies of women with thalassemia major[45]. Cardiac, hepatic and endocrine function should therefore be monitored carefully during pregnancy and in the postpartum period[46]. Delivery by Cesarean section may be planned prior to the due date, usually at between 37 and 38 weeks gestation to reduce the risk of complications for the mother, and to enable delivery to take place at a time when all necessary support services are available[47].

Sickle cell disease. Mothers with sickle cell disease are at increased risk of spontaneous abortion and stillbirth[48]. Severe anemia in pregnancy (hemoglobin <60–70% of the levels in unaffected women) is treated with blood transfusion. Trials of prophylactic transfusions to improve outcomes of pregnancy have not been conclusive[49].

Congenital heart disease.   Due to the success in treating congenital heart defects, around 1–3% of pregnancies may be complicated by a cardiac condition in the mother[50]. All women who have a history of heart defect, or experience cardiac problems during pregnancy, should be under the care of a cardiologist as well as an obstetrician during pregnancy. Congenital heart disease due to a genetic condition may not be treated any differently than that which occurs sporadically, however, there may be additional health factors to be considered in women who have a genetic condition affecting organs outside the cardiovascular system. For example, a woman with heart disease due to a chromosome 22q microdeletion may have learning difficulties and problems with immunity. Prophylactic antibiotics are often considered for use during labor. Whilst vaginal delivery is recommended for many conditions, a Cesarean section may be the best option in a woman who is already cyanosed and who is being delivered prematurely, and for those women with Marfan syndrome. Specific guidance is available on the management of a woman with a congenital heart defect[50].

7.2.6 *Skeletal conditions*

Women who have a genetic condition that affects the skeleton should be assessed to ensure that appropriate arrangements are made for the management of the pregnancy. Skeletal abnormalities may cause difficulties during birth, because of changes to the birth canal, and mothers may also experience pain and restricted mobility during pregnancy due to the unusual pressure on the skeleton. Mothers with achondroplasia may also be at risk of complications during pregnancy because the fetus is developing in an abdominal cavity that is shorter than usual. In addition, if both parents have achondroplasia, and the fetus inherits two mutated copies of a particular gene, this may be fatal, causing stillbirth[51].

CASE EXAMPLE   LYDIA AND JONNY

Lydia was a 32-year-old woman with achondroplasia. She and her partner Jonny, who also had achondroplasia, both wanted a large family. When Lydia became pregnant, her midwife was keen to make the pregnancy as normal as possible for them. Both Lydia and Jonny felt they had a very good quality of life and were not particularly concerned about having a child with achondroplasia. In fact, they joked about wanting a child who would be able to look up to them! Because the midwife knew they would not consider termination of pregnancy, she did not suggest a referral to the genetics service; she said she would refer Lydia to the obstetrician for discussion about the safest form of delivery. The couple decided against antenatal screening for Down syndrome, but wanted an anomaly scan to see if the fetus had inherited achondroplasia. When Lydia went for her scan at 19 weeks, it was discovered that the fetus had a lethal condition as a result of inheriting a mutation from both parents. The couple were given the option of terminating the pregnancy. As they were told the fetus could not survive until term, they opted to have a termination of pregnancy. As a result of genetic counseling after delivery, they became aware that in any future pregnancy the fetus would have a 25% chance of having the same lethal condition. While early referral to the genetic service would not have prevented the lethal condition in the fetus, Lydia and Jonny would have been prepared and would have had the opportunity to make decisions about testing earlier in the pregnancy. Three years later, they are still feeling traumatized by the loss of their son and have not wanted to start another pregnancy.

7.3 Spontaneous abortion (miscarriage)

Spontaneous abortion is thought to occur in about 10–15% of confirmed pregnancies. Unfortunately, women with a history of miscarriage are less likely to carry subsequent pregnancies to term because the underlying reason may have an impact in successive pregnancies. There are many causes of spontaneous abortion, these include:

- anatomical abnormality (e.g. bicornuate uterus)
- infection (e.g. herpes, cytomegalovirus or rubella)
- maternal hormonal imbalance (e.g. progesterone deficiency)
- endocrine dysfunction in the mother (e.g. poorly controlled diabetes)
- maternal immunological abnormality (e.g. systemic lupus erythematosis)

Beside these causes, an unbalanced chromosome arrangement in the fetus is believed to be the cause of up to 50% of spontaneous abortions[52]. This explains why the percentage of pregnancies that spontaneously abort increases with maternal age[53], as an unbalanced fetal chromosome arrangement is increasingly likely to occur as the mother grows older (see *Section 4.2* for further explanation).

In any pregnancy, there is a risk that the fetus will have an unbalanced chromosome arrangement, but many of these pregnancies result in spontaneous abortion even before the mother is aware that she has conceived. The chromosome imbalance may occur sporadically; less frequently it is inherited from a parent with a chromosome translocation.

Because most cases of chromosomal imbalance in a fetus occur sporadically, the parents have a low risk of the same problem occurring for a second time. Thus a mother who has conceived one child with a chromosomal abnormality will usually have less than a 1% chance of having another child with that condition. The exception to this general rule occurs when a parent has a balanced chromosome rearrangement.

As a cause of spontaneous abortion, a balanced translocation is usually not suspected until there have been at least two, but usually three, pregnancies lost in this way. After recurrent abortion, it is good practice to investigate the chromosome patterns of both parents. If one of the parents has a balanced translocation or rearrangement, there will usually be at least a 50% chance that in each pregnancy the fetus will inherit a balanced chromosome arrangement and will therefore develop normally. However, the precise risk figure depends on the nature of the parental rearrangement and, in each individual case, information should be sought from the cytogeneticist or genetic counselor about the risks to the particular couple, and whether prenatal diagnosis is advised in future pregnancies.

Whilst many parents find losing a pregnancy very distressing, some are able to rationalize it by concluding that the fetus was not developing normally and that the abortion was 'nature's way' of preventing the birth of an abnormal child. Whilst this thought may not lessen their sense of loss, it may help them to make sense of what has happened. Many parents express their sense of frustration and hurt that their friends or family do not regard the expected baby as 'real' and therefore minimize the loss, or ignore it altogether.

KEY PRACTICE POINT

After a couple have experienced a spontaneous abortion, explore with them the meaning of the miscarriage to them. For some, it will be 'just one of those things', for others a deeply felt loss. If they have named the baby, use the given name and acknowledge the reality of the loss.

CASE EXAMPLE **TERRY AND ROSE**

Terry and Rose were referred to the genetic service after experiencing three miscarriages. Their family doctor had taken a blood sample for karyotyping after the loss of the third pregnancy, and Terry was found to have a balanced translocation of chromosomes 2 and 6.

At first, the couple were pleased to have discovered the cause of their failure to carry a pregnancy to term, and they were encouraged when told there was a 50% chance of success in each pregnancy.

Terry was one of four children. His brothers and sister were offered chromosome analysis, as were his parents. Terry's mother had four normal pregnancies with no spontaneous abortions, so it seemed unlikely either of his parents carried the translocation.

However, Terry's father was found to carry the same translocation. Although Terry and Rose acknowledged that this meant they were likely to have a live baby, they also felt very angry that they had been so unlucky in losing three pregnancies, when Terry's parents had lost none. One of Terry's brothers was also found to carry the translocation.

Rose became pregnant again, and aborted at 6 weeks gestation. The couple then started to consider other reproductive options, as they felt that each miscarriage was devastating and they could not bear any more emotional strain. Whilst awaiting an appointment at the reproductive medicine clinic, Rose again became pregnant, only to miscarry a fifth pregnancy.

At this stage, the risk figure of 50% seemed inaccurate to them – how could they lose five pregnancies in a row?

A letter came from the reproductive medicine clinic, stating they would need to discuss the options fully before treatment was offered. Both partners were very upset, feeling this cast doubts on their ability to decide the best course of action for themselves and belittled the distress they had suffered. They cancelled the appointment.

When Rose became pregnant for the sixth time they hardly dared to hope. However, this time the pregnancy proceeded normally. They discussed prenatal diagnosis, but decided against an invasive procedure as they did not want to take any risk of losing a normal pregnancy due to complications of amniocentesis. They opted for high resolution ultrasound but were adamant that even if an abnormality was found they would not wish to terminate the pregnancy.

Terry and Rose had a normal baby girl at term. They have decided not to try and increase the family as they are too fearful of the pain of another miscarriage.

7.4 Down syndrome (trisomy 21)

Down syndrome occurs when an embryo has developed with an additional copy of chromosome 21. This usually occurs sporadically, because one gamete (either the ovum or the sperm) has been formed with two copies of chromosome 21, rather than the normal single copy. The recurrence risk is therefore usually low. Before advising parents, it is important to check the report of the chromosomal structure of the affected child. If the result shows that the child inherited a full additional copy of chromosome 21, (i.e. 47,XX,+21 or 47,XY,+21) then it is highly likely to have occurred sporadically. In this case, the risk for future pregnancies for this couple will be 1% or twice the mother's age-related risk, whichever is higher. Table 7.1 shows age-related risks for sporadic Down syndrome.

If, however, the chromosome result shows the child with Down syndrome had a translocation, the parents' chromosomes should be studied to ascertain whether one of them carries a Robertsonian translocation, as this would increase their chances of having a second child with a chromosomal abnormality. For example, if the father has a Robertsonian translocation, one of his copies of chromosome 14 will be attached to one copy of chromosome 21. If the sperm contains the translocated copy of 14 (with 21 attached) and a single copy of chromosome 21, the fetus will inherit two copies of chromosome 21 from the father and one from the mother. This could recur in a future pregnancy.

Table 7.1. Maternal age-related risk table for Down syndrome (live births)[40]

Age of mother at time of baby's birth	Risk of baby affected with Down syndrome
15 years	1 in 1580
20 years	1 in 1530
25 years	1 in 1350
30 years	1 in 901
35 years	1 in 385
37 years	1 in 240
39 years	1 in 145
41 years	1 in 85
43 years	1 in 49
45 years	1 in 28
47 years	1 in 15
49 years	1 in 8

KEY PRACTICE POINT

When advising a couple about the recurrence risk for Down syndrome, the chromosome pattern of the child with Down syndrome should be checked. If it is not available (e.g. because the child was stillborn or records were not kept), the parental chromosomes should be studied to ensure that neither parent carries a Robertsonian translocation.

Screening tests for Down syndrome are now offered to pregnant women in many countries and these will be discussed in the next section.

7.5 Antenatal screening

Screening test is the term used for any test where the result provides an *indication* of the level of risk in a particular pregnancy, whereas a diagnostic test (such as fetal karyotype after amniocentesis or chorionic villus sampling) usually provides the parents with a *definite* result. Antenatal screening of the fetus can be performed for a range of conditions, including chromosomal abnormalities (such as trisomy) and physical structural abnormalities (such as neural tube defect or congenital heart disease). Screening may be offered using either biochemical markers or ultrasound, or a combination of both. All healthcare professionals who come into contact with a pregnant couple should be aware of the types of antenatal screening options they may be offered. The majority of screening tests are carried out in women who are not at increased risk (i.e. general population risk) and in whom any abnormality found would not have been predicted because of previous family or medical history.

The midwife has a particular responsibility when discussing choices for routine antenatal screening or diagnosis to ensure that the woman is given enough information to allow her to make a truly informed choice. There are guidelines for offering antenatal screening tests, such as those set by the Council of Europe[54] and the UK National Screening Committee[55]. These state that the information that should be provided to women considering antenatal screening must include the type of screening offered, information that the screening tests are optional, the limitations of the screening tests, false positive and false negative rates, the types of diagnostic tests that will be offered if the fetus is found to be at high risk, and the way in which parents will be told of the results. However, studies have shown that in many settings the screening tests might be regarded as 'routine' by both professionals and parents[56]. This leads to parents being unaware they have a choice and precludes informed decision making. This issue is going to become even more relevant as screening for abnormality becomes increasingly part of routine antenatal care. It is also important to recognize that if a high-risk screening result is obtained, couples will then be placed in a situation where they will be offered diagnostic tests and may eventually be offered the option of terminating an affected pregnancy. While this is a valid choice for them to be offered, it is essential that the full consequences of screening be explored with a pregnant couple in order that they can make the choice that best fits their own beliefs, values and particular circumstances.

In any situation, the offer of a screening or diagnostic test should not be conditional on the parents agreeing to termination if the fetus is found to be abnormal. That decision remains with the parents, and some may choose to continue with a pregnancy. However, they should be aware that some tests are invasive, and as such carry a risk to the fetus. If the results of the test would not affect their continuing with the pregnancy, taking that risk may not be justified.

7.5.1 *Antenatal screening for Down syndrome*

In many countries, screening for Down syndrome is now being offered to all pregnant women as part of their antenatal care. The screening test result provides an indication of the level of risk for the fetus in a particular pregnancy, rather than a definite diagnosis, and therefore both false negative and false positive results are possible[57].

Parents whose fetus is assessed as having a significant chance of being affected with Down syndrome are offered invasive diagnostic testing (amniocentesis or chorionic villus sampling). Typically in the UK, the threshold for offering invasive testing is a chance of Down syndrome equal to or greater than 1 in 250[57]. Screening programs in the UK currently focus on detecting Down syndrome. It is known that increasing maternal age leads to a higher risk of having a baby with Down syndrome. Amniocentesis may be offered to all women who will be over a certain age at the birth of the baby, normally 35 or 37, depending on the policy of individual health districts. However, even though an individual's risk of having a baby with Down syndrome is low, the majority of pregnancies occur in women under the age of 35, and so most babies born with Down syndrome will have mothers aged less than 35 years. Various screening methods[58] involving biochemical testing of the mother's blood and ultrasound scanning have been developed in an attempt to identify individual women whose pregnancy may be at increased risk. These include:

First trimester
- nuchal translucency measurement by ultrasound
- double test on maternal serum – PAPP-A (pregnancy-associated plasma protein A) and HCG (human chorionic gonadotrophin)
- combined nuchal translucency and double test

Second trimester
- double test on maternal serum – AFP (alpha fetoprotein) and HCG
- triple test on maternal serum – AFP, HCG and uE3 (unconjugated oestriol)
- quadruple test on maternal serum – AFP, HCG, uE3, inhibin A

The *integrated test* involves testing in both first and second trimester
- nuchal translucency and PAPP-A in first trimester
- quadruple test in second trimester

However, these tests only provide an estimate of the chance the fetus will have Down syndrome, rather than a definitive result. If the risk is greater than 1 in 250 (this threshold may vary according to the policy in the maternity unit), the mother is usually offered a test to check the karyotype of the fetus. Although the purpose of screening is to detect Down syndrome, the biochemical markers studied in maternal serum may be altered by other fetal abnormalities and the diagnosis of a completely unexpected abnormality may be made. The serum screening test result provides the parents with more information on which to base decisions about definitive testing, but the majority of those who have a serum screening result in the 'high risk' category will have a normal fetal karyotype (a false positive serum screening result). It must also be remembered that a serum screening result in the 'low risk' category does not rule out the possibility that the fetus does have Down syndrome (a false negative serum screening result). Increasingly, women are being offered nuchal translucency measurement as an alternative to serum screening. At the end of the first trimester a measurement is made of the fluid-filled space at the back of the neck. An unusually large measurement may indicate a fetus with Down syndrome. The integrated test has been shown to be the most effective method of screening for Down syndrome for women who present in the first trimester[59].

Development of new techniques, such as FISH and QfPCR, have meant that a rapid test can be offered for trisomies (see *Chapter 4*) with the result being available within 48 hours[60]. In some centers this is now the preferred diagnostic test in the Down syndrome screening program, and a full karyotype test is not offered unless there are other indications such as a nuchal thickness of greater than 3 mm or other scan abnormalities. It is essential that practitioners involved in caring for pregnant women are aware of the policy in their area.

New techniques for extracting and analyzing free fetal cells from a maternal blood sample have been developed. The analysis of free fetal DNA for rhesus incompatibility and sex determination is moving into routine practice.

Methods for determining the karyotype are also being developed and if they are successful may give couples the option of knowing the definitive karyotype of their expected baby without the risk of invasive tests.

7.5.2 *Ultrasound scanning*

Ultrasonography is now a routine part of most women's antenatal care. It should be emphasized that the purpose of scanning is to detect abnormality and not to provide reassurance of a normal pregnancy, although the outcome is normal in most routine scanning. The sensitivity of the ultrasound scan at detecting abnormality will depend on the stage of pregnancy and the nature of the abnormality. For example, a detailed scan at about 18 weeks gestation will detect more than 95% of babies with a neural tube defect, but only 30–50% of those with major heart abnormalities. If the pregnancy is at a higher risk of a heart abnormality, detailed specialist cardiac scanning can be offered at a specialist unit. A family history of a genetic disorder or congenital abnormality may indicate the need for a higher level of scanning than that which is routinely offered. Early scanning can be useful for dating purposes and may detect gross abnormalities such as anencephaly, however, the early dating scan is not a substitute for a later anomaly scan.

Scanning may detect abnormalities that are difficult to interpret, and further more invasive testing may be required. Certain structural markers such as specific congenital abnormalities (e.g. heart defect, renal abnormality or skeletal abnormality) may be an indication for chromosome analysis of the baby.

Recent work on this topic has shown that many women do not appreciate that an ultrasound scan is a type of screening test and that informed consent is therefore not always obtained[61]. Both midwives and ultrasonographers have a duty to ensure pregnant women who agree to a scan are aware that they are consenting to a screening test that may detect fetal abnormalities.

7.6 Antenatal testing techniques

Diagnostic testing of the fetus may be performed when the fetus is known to be at high risk, due to indicative family history or a high-risk screening result. Samples of blood or cells for testing are obtained by amniocentesis, chorionic villus sampling or, occasionally, **cordocentesis**. However, new non-invasive techniques involve using free fetal DNA or mRNA from maternal serum; this type of testing is only available for use in fetal sexing and for a small number of other conditions at present. In some cases, where there are clear anatomical changes, diagnosis of a genetic or congenital condition is possible using ultrasound scanning. Details of the methods and use of invasive and non-invasive techniques are provided below.

Couples that choose to continue with a pregnancy when the fetus has been diagnosed as having abnormalities or health problems require specific support from the midwifery team. Delivery may be planned in a center where access to surgical teams or specialist care is available. Routine care may be altered during labor, as fetal monitoring might not be appropriate if the condition is lethal. The method of delivery should also be planned as a Cesarean section delivery for a mother whose child will not survive would probably not be in the best interests of the mother.

If a couple choose to terminate a pregnancy, this is usually done via suction evacuation of the uterus under general anesthetic before 12–14 weeks gestation. After that time, labor is induced, often by the use of prostaglandin pessaries and intravenous oxytocin. As the cervix is usually firm, labor often lasts many hours, even several days. Sensitive support for both parents and appropriate analgesia for the mother are imperative.

7.6.1 Amniocentesis

Amniocentesis is usually performed at around 16 weeks gestation. It is normally offered to women who have an increased risk of a baby with a chromosome abnormality. This may be because of the mother's age or because other screening tests or the scan may suggest the pregnancy is at some risk. The amniotic fluid contains cells that are sloughed off the baby's skin, urinary tract and lungs. These cells can be cultured and a karyotype performed. In a pregnancy that may be at risk of rhesus disease, analysis of the bilirubin content of the amniotic fluid is used to assess the status of the baby. Amniocentesis can also be used to withdraw amniotic fluid for biochemical testing (for some specific metabolic conditions), or for viral studies if fetal infection is suspected. The test is carried out under ultrasound guidance and a full bladder is necessary. Local anesthetic is injected into the skin of the abdomen and a fine needle is passed through the skin into the uterus and the amniotic cavity (*Figure 7.2*). A small amount of fluid is withdrawn into a

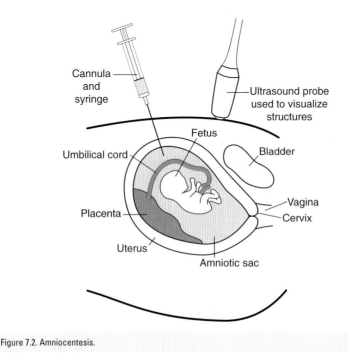

Figure 7.2. Amniocentesis.

syringe and the needle removed. The test is normally performed in the outpatient clinic.

The time taken for the results will depend on local circumstances, but is normally at least 7 days. The result is a full karyotype, which will show other abnormalities of chromosome number and structure in addition to Down syndrome. The implications of these other abnormalities may not be clear or may require expert interpretation. Some of them, such as abnormalities of the sex chromosomes, may not be as significant as Down syndrome. Amniocentesis has a risk of causing a miscarriage of between 0.5% and 1%, although the risks may vary according to the operator.

7.6.2 *Chorionic villus sampling or biopsy*

Chorionic villus sampling (CVS) is the method of choice for obtaining a sample for fetal DNA analysis, as DNA can be extracted from the chorionic villi more easily than from the fetal skin cells. The chorionic villi are the part of the placenta that attaches into the wall of the uterus. Since the placenta and the fetus arise from the same embryo they essentially share the same genetic and chromosomal material. CVS can also be used to obtain a sample of tissue that can be used for karyotyping.

The main advantage of CVS is that it is performed at about 10–12 weeks gestation and the early diagnosis is preferred by many women. The disadvantage is that it is considered to have a higher rate of miscarriage than amniocentesis, although this has been shown not to be the case in some centers with very experienced operators[62]. The exact miscarriage risk is difficult to determine since miscarriage is relatively common in early pregnancy. Individual centers usually maintain their own follow-up and will be able to quote a risk for their own center, which is normally in the region of 1–3%. There has also been a concern about a risk of limb abnormality with CVS; it is thought currently that this is related to the timing of the CVS, and for this reason the test is not performed earlier than 10 weeks gestation[63].

CVS is normally performed through the abdomen (*Figure 7.3*) in the same way as amniocentesis. It can also be done by inserting a fine cannula into the uterus, through the vagina and cervix. The result will normally take about a week. A result can be generated in 24–48 hours without culturing the cells. This analysis will not be at the same level of detail as a result from a culture and is more prone to error.

Whilst testing techniques have improved, and options are undoubtedly greater, the decision to terminate a pregnancy is difficult in any family. However, the family may be more certain that their decision was right for them when the outcome of the pregnancy is known with greater accuracy.

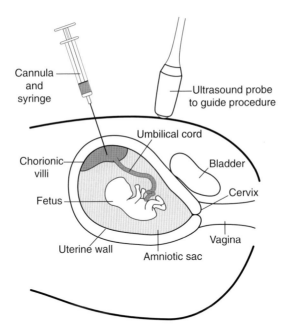

Figure 7.3. Chorionic villus sampling.

Harding Family

Referral letter

RE: Sarah Smith

This delightful 28-year-old patient of mine is unexpectedly pregnant. Her father was diagnosed with Huntington disease some years ago. Sarah is aware that a test for this is possible but has always said she would not want to know herself. Obviously the pregnancy may change the picture. Please see and advise.

Sarah was offered an urgent appointment with the genetic team and an ultrasound dating scan arranged. Sarah came to the appointment with her partner Nick and with her older sister Lauren. The genetic counselor realised that she had met Lauren in the past when the diagnosis in her father had been made. At that time Sarah was doing her A levels and had not wanted to be seen in the genetics department. The family file was reviewed and it became clear that the family had been known to the genetics department for many years. Various different members had been seen in the past and DNA samples had been collected for linkage studies (see Section 4.7.2; prior to identification of the gene mutation, linkage studies allowed some people to have predictive tests).

The genetic counselor asked Sarah about her family tree (Figure 7.4) in order to allow her to talk about what Huntington disease meant to her. Sarah was well informed and was very sure that she did not want to know if she had the gene; she felt she would not be able to cope with living with the knowledge that she was going to develop Huntington disease. She and Nick were also sure that they did not want to pass the gene on to the current pregnancy which they had already decided that they wanted to continue if possible. The dating scan had shown that Sarah was eight weeks pregnant.

The counselor discussed the options that were available to Sarah and Nick:

(i)   have a termination of the pregnancy on the basis it was unplanned

(ii)   continue with the pregnancy on the basis it was at 25% risk

(iii)   have a predictive test for Sarah and then test the fetus if she should prove to have the gene

(iv)   have an **exclusion test** on the pregnancy; this was possible because the family was already known to the department and some linkage analysis had already been done

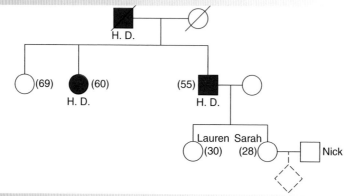

Figure 7.4. Family tree.

Sarah did not want to take the risk of continuing without testing, as she said she didn't wish to 'Put another person through what I'm going through now'. Nor did she want to know at this time if she had the gene. Gene testing would have been a very rushed procedure because of the need to get the results back in order to do a CVS at ten weeks if the predictive test on Sarah showed that she had the gene.

Sarah decided on an exclusion test using linked markers. Linkage results using markers closely linked to the Huntington gene had shown that her father had inherited different genetic markers from his parents. In the past Sarah's mother had also given a DNA sample and the results had shown that she had different genetic markers at the HD locus from her husband. This means that in Sarah it was possible to distinguish between the maternal and paternal markers (Figure 7.5).

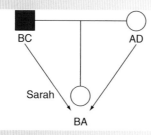

Figure 7.5. Linkage results.

In Sarah the marker A inherited from her mother would not be linked to the HD gene; if this marker was passed on to the fetus it would be at low risk. In her father it is not known if the marker B or C is linked to the HD gene (remember that he will have one normal gene and one HD gene). However, because marker B is inherited from her affected parent, if this marker is passed on to the fetus it will be at the same risk as Sarah – 50%. Therefore it would be possible to tell if the pregnancy was at low risk or high risk.

The counselor spent some time discussing what Sarah and Nick would do if the pregnancy was at high risk. If the pregnancy continued and Sarah then developed HD, the baby would have been shown to have inherited the gene, because it would then be known that marker B was linked to the HD gene in Sarah's father. This would be a very difficult situation for that child to be in and not at all desirable. It was also important for Sarah and Nick to understand that if the pregnancy was high risk and was terminated and Sarah was then shown not to have the gene for HD, then they would have terminated a healthy baby.

Sarah and Nick still thought that they would have the test and would terminate a pregnancy at high risk. In order to see if the test was possible, a DNA sample was needed from Nick. For the linkage to be informative for the pregnancy it has to be possible to distinguish between the markers that the fetus had inherited from Sarah and from Nick. The linkage test would also have a small error rate because of recombination. It would theoretically be possible for the markers to cross over during meiosis, even though they are tightly linked to the HD locus.

Because Sarah was eight weeks pregnant, they were given another appointment in one week's time to discuss all the results and go over the details of exclusion testing again. The results of the DNA typing are shown in Figure 7.6, together with the possible outcomes for the pregnancy.

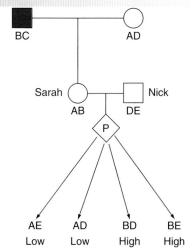

Figure 7.6. Possible linkage results.

Nick and Sarah came to the appointment, on their own this time. They were very clear about their decision, which was to go ahead with testing. A CVS was booked for ten weeks of gestation. Sarah decided that she wanted to be telephoned at home with the result in the evening, when they both would be home from work, and this was agreed.

A week after the CVS was done the DNA result came through. It showed that the pregnancy was at low risk. Sarah and Nick were delighted and continued with the pregnancy. They wanted to be seen again after the baby was born to go over what had happened and a follow-up appointment was arranged. As the conversation with the genetic counselor was ending, Sarah mentioned that she was very worried about Lauren. She had become anxious and depressed and seemed to be a bit clumsy, but would not talk about it or see any one. They agreed to talk about this again at the follow-up appointment.

KEY PRACTICE POINT

DNA analysis for prenatal diagnosis may require some work to be done in the molecular genetics laboratory before it is possible to offer a test. It is essential that the genetics laboratory, the clinical genetics team, and the obstetric and midwifery team, liaise closely when such testing is being considered. Early referral (before pregnancy if possible) is also essential.

7.6.3 *Cordocentesis*

Occasionally it may be desirable to sample some blood from the fetus. The sample is taken from the umbilical cord and can be taken after 16 weeks of gestation (*Figure 7.7*). It can be used as a source of cells for karyotyping or for direct analysis of the blood, e.g. for an assessment of anemia. The test has a miscarriage risk of approximately 5%.

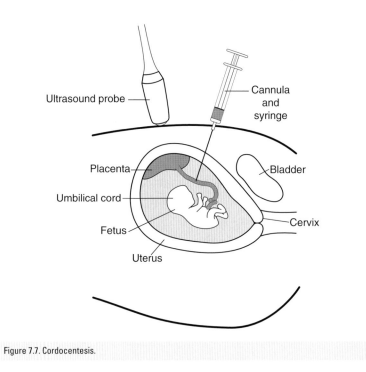

Figure 7.7. Cordocentesis.

7.6.4 *Non-invasive techniques for testing fetal material*

There are several methods that have been developed to enable testing of fetal material without the need for an invasive procedure such as amniocentesis or CVS[64]. These techniques are possible due to the crossover of fetal cells into the maternal circulation via the placenta. Testing is carried out using a maternal blood sample.

Some researchers have used retrieved fetal cells (cytotrophoblasts that originate in the placenta) from the maternal blood, but there are a comparatively small number of fetal cells in the mother's circulation, which presents a practical difficulty[65]. Cell-free fetal DNA from the cytotrophoblasts is also present in the maternal circulation, and can be used for testing in some conditions by examining the alleles from the father[66]. Fetal DNA comprises about 3–6% of DNA in the mother's blood supply[65], and is quickly cleared after delivery so that the DNA from one baby is not present in subsequent pregnancies. Messenger RNA from the fetus has been tested to detect trisomy 21 by using **single nucleotide polymorphisms (SNPs)** to compare the ratio of alleles; in a fetus with trisomy 21 there will be twice as many of one allele compared to the other. As mentioned before, use of these techniques for fetal sexing and rhesus typing is becoming routine, and techniques for detecting Down syndrome and other aneuploidies are being developed[67]. Many of these techniques still require further evaluation for general clinical use.

7.7 Examination of the neonate

It is essential that any newborn is examined by the midwife or doctor to detect any unusual or abnormal features at birth. Whilst this is important for a healthy infant, the results of the examination assume greater significance if the baby is stillborn or dies soon after birth. Couples who have lost a child around the time of birth are understandably shocked and distressed, and a future pregnancy may well be the furthest thought from their minds. However, when they begin to consider another pregnancy, one of their main concerns will be the possibility of recurrence.

It is impossible to offer accurate information about the recurrence risk without detailed records of the baby who did not survive. It is therefore vital that, whatever the outlook of the parents at the time of birth, the midwife examines the baby thoroughly and carefully documents any unusual features (*Figure 7.8*). It is equally important to *document* normal findings, as this enables the genetic counselor to give a more informed opinion about the causes of death and chance of similar events occurring in the future.

7.8 Post-mortem examination of a neonate

The subject of the post-mortem examination of the baby after a stillbirth or **neonatal death** is a sensitive one. Pressure or coercion should certainly never be applied to induce the parents to consent against their will. However, the decision should be an informed one, and therefore parents need information about the limitations on advice for the future if a post-mortem is not conducted. The post-mortem examination provides accurate information about the cause of death and a detailed assessment of any external and internal abnormalities. Both are usually necessary for a genetic risk assessment to be made.

Suggested checklist of features for examination of baby		
Gestational age		
Length		
Weight		
OFC		
	Head	Shape
		Fontanelles
	Hair	Texture
		Color
		Quantity
Face		
	Eyes	Brows
		Lashes
		Irides
		Lens
	Mouth	Size
		Shape
		Lips
		Palate
	Nose	Shape
		Bridge
		Nares
	Philtrum	
Mid-face		
	Jaw	
	Ears	Position
		Size
		Shape
Chest		
	Abdomen	Herniae
		Genitalia
		Testes
Limbs		
	Hands	Nails
		Fingers
		Creases
		Size
	Feet	Nails
		Toes
		Hallux
		Creases
		Size
	Skin	Unusual patterns
		Birthmarks
		Skin tags

Figure 7.8. Suggested checklist for the neonatal examination.

If the parents do not wish to consent to a post-mortem, good quality photographs of the baby should be taken for the medical records, if possible by a medical photographer. These should include pictures of any abnormal features, the face, hands and feet. The parents may also consent to an external physical examination by a pathologist and/or X-rays. In addition, cord blood, venous blood or a skin sample can be sent for chromosome analysis. It is often possible to culture cells from the skin sample even if the baby is stillborn, although the culture is not likely to be successful if the fetus is significantly macerated. Amniocentesis performed before a termination of pregnancy may give the best opportunity for chromosome analysis on the fetus.

After spontaneous abortion or termination of pregnancy, products of conception can be sent for chromosome analysis in a container of normal saline or tissue culture medium.

KEY PRACTICE POINT

To obtain a karyotype from a stillborn child, a small sample of skin can be taken from the upper leg using a skin biopsy punch or a small scalpel blade. The tissue should then be placed in tissue culture medium. Samples for karyotyping should NEVER be placed in formalin. The sample needs to be sent to the cytogenetics laboratory as a matter of urgency as delay lessens the chance that the culture will grow adequately.

Following a stillbirth, neonatal death, or termination of pregnancy for fetal abnormality, parents may be reluctant to look at their baby, particularly if they are aware of congenital abnormalities. In fact, the parents may imagine features that are much more frightening than the actuality. In our experience the decision not to see the baby is often deeply regretted later. Skillful reassurance from the midwife may encourage the parents to see their baby, thus reducing later regrets and enabling the parents to grieve more appropriately. Dressing the baby and wrapping him or her in a blanket will enable the parents to view their son or daughter in their own time if they wish to do so. Many parents are reassured by the normality of the majority of the features, it should be remembered that even babies with gross abnormalities such an anencephaly have a normal trunk, limbs, hands and feet. If the parents do not wish to see their baby, consent should be sought to take some photographs. These can be kept securely in the notes and requested by the parents later. Handprints, footprints, or any item connected with the baby such as identity bands may be treasured by the parents. Such momentos help to reinforce the reality of the baby's existence, and may be helpful to the parents as they mourn.

7.9 Conclusion

In this chapter, we have provided some guidelines for the care of a mother who has a genetic condition, for a couple requesting genetic testing during pregnancy, and the examination of a neonate. The discussion questions at the end of this chapter are designed to help the reader think about the psychological issues in more depth. The next chapter of the book deals with genetic problems that may become obvious during infancy.

Test yourself

Q1. Sally was a 22-year-old woman, pregnant for the first time. The ultrasound scan performed at 18 weeks showed that the fetus had a heart defect, and an amniocentesis was carried out. Down syndrome was diagnosed in the fetus. Sally's partner was adamant he could not cope with an abnormal child and they decided to have the pregnancy terminated at 22 weeks. Sally was afraid to see the baby, whom she dreaded would look grossly abnormal.

How can midwives or nurses present at the delivery of a baby with abnormalities discuss the baby's features realistically without creating fear in the parent? What terms could be used?

Q2. A woman who is 10 weeks pregnant is offered screening for Down syndrome. She refuses to listen to any explanation of the test, saying she just wants any test that helps ensure her baby is healthy. How can the professional involved ensure the woman is giving informed consent?

Q3. The parents of a stillborn baby with multiple abnormalities do not consent to a post-mortem. What can the professional do to ensure that information about the baby is recorded?

Further resources

www.adhb.govt.nz/newborn/Education/Teaching/5thYearsNewborn
Exam.htm – New Zealand Government information on examination of the newborn. *Detailed information on examination of the newborn.*
www.antenataltesting.info/ – AnSWeR. *Antenatal screening web resource for parents.*
www.healthtalkonline.org/Pregnancy_children/ – Health Talk Online. *Stories from parents on their experience of pregnancy, screening, genetic testing and ending a pregnancy because of fetal abnormality.*
www.healthtalkonline.org/Pregnancy_children/Antenatal_Screening – Health Talk Online – antenatal screening. *True stories from women about their experiences of antenatal screening.*

www.healthtalkonline.org/Pregnancy_children/Ending_a_pregnancy_for_
fetal_abnormality – Health Talk Online – termination for fetal
abnormality. *True stories from women who have undergone termination for fetal
abnormality.*

www.library.nhs.uk/screening/SearchResults.aspx?catID=1328 – National
Library for Health. *Antenatal screening section.*

www.screening.nhs.uk/cpd/webfolder/resources/ANS_workbook_2.html –
Screening Choices Toolbox. *Antenatal screening information for professionals.*

8 Infancy

8.1 Introduction

It is important for the practitioner to remember that despite the majority of pregnancies ending with the birth of an apparently healthy child, in approximately 3% of pregnancies the baby is born with a significant congenital abnormality or disease. In addition, neonatal screening programs may detect a genetic condition in an apparently healthy neonate.

The health professional at this time needs to be able to give and interpret accurate information, taking into account the distress and shock of the parents and making an assessment of their particular needs. There may be an urgent medical need to define the diagnosis so that treatment decisions can be made and information provided about the prognosis. For example, if the baby has a chromosomal abnormality that is not consistent with survival beyond several days or weeks, the decision might be made by the parents and health professionals to avoid interventions that would be painful or distressing to the baby. However, there may be considerable uncertainty about a diagnosis and it is possible that one will not be made at this time, because important signs and symptoms of the condition may not yet be apparent. It is very understandable that parents will be searching for a diagnosis that explains the condition of their child, and the lack of certainty at this time can be very difficult. One important role of the health professional is to help the family to focus on the needs of the child, which they have some power to address, rather than the actual diagnosis.

In this chapter we will describe some of the more common congenital abnormalities, discuss neonatal screening programs and describe the possible diagnostic pathways for babies with chromosome abnormalities and neurological problems.

For the practitioner to work in partnership with the parents and the medical team, he or she needs to be informed and to understand the process of diagnosis and management of a genetic condition. In this way they can effectively care for the baby and the family as they come to terms with the difficulties they may be facing.

8.2 Congenital abnormalities

A congenital abnormality can be described as an alteration in the normal pattern of structural development, which is present at birth. Congenital abnormalities may be characterized according to the possible mechanism that caused them, whether they are isolated or multiple and whether they occur in a known pattern.

CATEGORIES OF BIRTH DEFECTS

Malformation: a specific primary alteration in development, e.g. cardiac defect or neural tube defect.

Deformation: an abnormal development of a structure caused by outside forces, e.g. talipes caused by oligohydramnios.

Disruption: alteration of normally formed tissue, e.g. amniotic bands causing limb amputations.

PATTERNS OF BIRTH DEFECTS

Isolated: involving a single organ system, e.g. isolated cleft palate.

Association: the non-random association of groups of congenital anomalies in a relatively inconsistent manner, e.g. VACTERL association vertebral anomalies, anal atresia, cardiac anomalies, tracheo-oesophageal fistula, renal anomalies and limb defects.

Syndrome: a consistent pattern of defects between unrelated individuals, e.g. Down syndrome, velocardiofacial syndrome (see Case example – Amy), Cornelia de Lange syndrome.

8.2.1 *Cleft lip and palate*

About 1 in 500 to 1 in 1000 children are born with a cleft lip or palate. Although isolated cleft lip and/or palate are essentially treatable with surgery, parents can be concerned about the possibility of having a child with similar problems in the future.

In order to give accurate recurrence risks, a careful examination must be made to exclude other anomalies that may indicate that the clefting is part of a syndrome rather than isolated malformation. Some examples of syndromes associated with cleft lip and/or palate are:

- Van der Woude syndrome (autosomal dominant – lip pits with cleft lip/palate)
- Stickler syndrome (autosomal dominant – hereditary arthro-ophthalmopathy)
- trisomy 13
- chromosome 22q microdeletion

Maternal contact with **teratogens** (such as anti-epileptic medication) can also be implicated in the formation of cleft lip/palate and should also be considered, since this may indicate the need for review of the management of a future pregnancy. However, some women have unstable epilepsy and there may be few choices about the medications. It is generally considered to be more dangerous for the mother and fetus (due to possible fetal hypoxia during fits) if the mother has uncontrolled epilepsy.

Studies have shown that cleft palate alone is a separate condition from cleft lip with or without cleft palate. Isolated cleft lip and/or palate are generally considered to be multifactorial/polygenic in etiology, although it is now thought that a proportion may be due to mutations in single genes. The empiric recurrence risks for future pregnancies after the birth of one affected child are between 2% and 4%. Obviously, if the clefting is due to a familial gene mutation that is present in a parent, the chances of recurrence in another child in the family are greater than if the event is sporadic or multi-factorial.

CASE EXAMPLE   AMY

Amy was born at term and was noted to have a cleft palate. In addition to this she had a very small jaw. This caused her problems in maintaining her airway and she required initial ventilation. The diagnosis of Pierre–Robin sequence was made (*Figure 8.1*). The small jaw seen in Pierre–Robin sequence is thought to be a result of the failure of the tongue to influence jaw development in the usual way. This is because the tongue lies on the roof of the mouth due to the cleft palate. Amy's mother Debbie was put in touch with the Pierre–Robin sequence support group. She received a lot of support through an internet bulletin board, where she was able to ask questions of other parents and find out that her experience was not unique. Although Debbie initially had a lot of problems feeding Amy, she took the advice of other mothers and adapted her feeding techniques to suit Amy better.

(a)   (b)

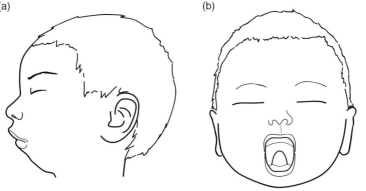

Figure 8.1. Pierre–Robin sequence showing (a) the typical small mandible and (b) the 'U'-shaped cleft palate (these may also be 'V'-shaped).

The prognosis for an infant with Pierre–Robin sequence is good with careful management, and the recurrence risk for future pregnancies is generally low. Amy's mother was reassured by this, as her cousin Faye was pregnant and due to have her baby at any time.

When Faye's baby was born she was noted to have a cleft uvula, bilateral dislocated hips and large round eyes. The geneticist who saw the family at that time found out that several members of the family were very short sighted and that some of them had had detached retinas. In addition, some members of the family had arthritis of the hips and knees. The geneticist made the diagnosis of Stickler syndrome. This is an autosomal dominant syndrome with cleft palate, high myopia with retinal detachment, and arthropathy. The expression and penetrance is very variable. In addition, the condition is **heterogeneous** with at least three genes having been identified, with many different mutations. All the genes identified code for collagen, a component of connective tissue.

After putting the family history together (*Figure 8.2*) it became clear that Faye and Debbie both had the gene mutation that causes Stickler syndrome. Faye had always worn glasses and at school was a bit 'double jointed', but had had no other health problems. Debbie felt that Faye and herself were obviously from the same family, they took after their grandfather and looked more like sisters than cousins, but Faye had no medical problems. Their grandfather had had a hip replacement in his 50s and had in fact gone blind suddenly which family said was due to shock in the war.

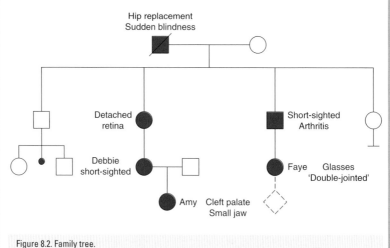

Figure 8.2. Family tree.

Because Stickler syndrome is an autosomal dominant condition, both Faye and Debbie would have a 50% chance of passing the gene on to any of their children. However, how the gene would be expressed in any individual child could not be predicted. Debbie asked if the gene was 'stronger' in her since she felt Amy had been quite severely affected. The different ways the gene affected people in the family is an example of variable penetrance and expression.

Apart from the way this diagnosis changed the information about prognosis and recurrence risks, it also has important implications for management. The children and other members of the family now see an ophthalmologist regularly for review so that any problems can be detected quickly and treated to reduce the risk of blindness.

KEY PRACTICE POINT

The practitioner should be able to distinguish between isolated anomalies and patterns that may be significant and then initiate the appropriate referral. Even seemingly unconnected abnormalities may be part of an overall pattern with variable expression.

8.2.2 *Neural tube defect*

The term neural tube defect (NTD) includes spina bifida, anencephaly, and any other defect that is a failure of closure of the neural tube. The incidence of spina bifida varies between countries, regions of countries, and also over time. Importantly, the campaign to encourage prospective mothers to take folic acid supplements has had an enormous impact on the incidence of the condition. For example, in Western Australia until 1996 around 2 children in every 1000 were born with a NTD. Since 1996, the figure has dropped to 1.3 children per 1000 births as a result of the folic acid campaign. Since spina bifida accounts for approximately half of all NTDs, this means the birth rate for spina bifida since 1996 has been between 0.5 and 0.7 per 1000 births.

As is the case with many other malformations (such as cleft palate), when seeing a family for genetic counseling it is important to distinguish between cases where the NTD is isolated and those where it forms part of a syndrome. The recurrence risk for isolated NTDs is approximately 4% but, as discussed in *Chapter 6*, this can be reduced by ensuring an adequate intake of folic acid.

It should be noted that spina bifida and anencephaly are probably part of the same spectrum and the recurrence risk includes the whole spectrum. This may make a difference to how a family will perceive the recurrence risk. For example, a couple may decide they would not terminate a pregnancy if the child had spina bifida but would not wish to go through a pregnancy where the fetus was affected with anencephaly and would therefore not survive. If that couple would find it difficult to terminate a pregnancy, they may decide not to have further children because of the chance of anencephaly.

Hydrocephalus is often associated with NTDs as a secondary consequence of disturbance of the circulation of the cerebro-spinal fluid. There is a rare form of X-linked hydrocephalus associated with mutations in the LCAM gene and hydrocephalus may also be part of other rare syndromes. Careful examination is needed to exclude NTDs before considering that a baby with hydrocephalus has one of these rare isolated forms.

8.2.3 *Gastroschisis*

Gastroschisis describes a failure of closure of the abdominal wall, which allows the intestines to protrude through the wall. There is no evidence that this is genetic and the recurrence risk is low. However, use of recreational drugs by the mother has been implicated in the malformation[68]. The maternal serum AFP levels will be raised due to the leakage of AFP from the fetus through the uncovered abdominal wall. Gastroschisis is often detected by ultrasound in the second trimester[69].

8.2.4 *Congenital heart defects*

The recurrence risk for isolated congenital heart defects (CHDs) varies according to the nature of the defect. With improvements in surgery, children who would not have survived in the past are now surviving to reproductive age. Adults who were born with a CHD may request information about the risks to their own children but, as yet, there is little empiric information on which to base a risk assessment. However, there are ample data on the risks when other first degree relatives, such as siblings, are affected and these can be used to guide genetic counseling.

Many chromosome abnormalities are associated with CHD and chromosome analysis should be considered if there are any other associated abnormalities. The identification of a microdeletion on the long arm of chromosome 22 that is associated with cono-truncal cardiac abnormalities has clarified the etiology in a subset of patients with those types of defects, and detailed chromosome analysis should be considered if appropriate. Microdeletions of 22q are found in more than half of children born with interrupted aortic arch or truncus arteriosus. Identification of such a deletion has implications for recurrence risk and also for the presence of associated abnormalities[70].

8.3 Chromosome abnormalities

If a baby is born with a combination of congenital abnormalities, a chromosome abnormality should be considered as a possible cause and chromosome analysis should normally be undertaken. As discussed in *Chapter 4*, karyotyping can be carried out at varying levels of detail. For example, a rapid karyotype reported in 24 hours may be sufficient to exclude trisomies such as Down syndrome or trisomy 18, but may not detect subtle deletions or rearrangements.

Studies of unselected newborn populations[71] show that approximately 1% of newborns had recognizable chromosome abnormalities, about three-quarters

The Singh Family

Baby Jahan Singh was born late one evening at 38 weeks gestation, after labor was induced because of suspected intrauterine growth retardation. His mother Maya had a normal vaginal delivery. Jahan's apgar score was 3 at 5 minutes, but had risen to 7 by 10 minutes. His weight at birth was 2.2 kg.

The initial physical examination revealed that Jahan had a cleft palate and he was admitted to the special care baby unit for the night. During the night he was noted to be jittery and serum calcium levels were taken. He was hypocalcemic. The pediatrician also detected a heart murmur and ordered an echocardiogram for the following day.

The next day a cardiac defect was diagnosed, but immediate treatment was not necessary. Jahan was stable and started breastfeeding with a plate in situ, although he tired easily and his feeds were supplemented by nasogastric feeds of expressed breast milk.

The pediatrician explained to Maya and Rajesh that Jahan's health problems were all due to a tiny change in one chromosome. Chromosome analysis had shown Jahan had a microdeletion of chromosome 22q. She told them that this could have occurred for the first time in Jahan, but might have been inherited from one side of the family. The family history indicated that because Rajit had some learning problems, which can be caused by genes on 22q, it seemed more likely it had originated in his side of the family. In addition, he had required speech therapy as a child and this could have been linked to a sub-mucous cleft palate. The pediatrician asked if the couple would consent to have blood taken for chromosome studies on them both, but as it would not help Jahan in any way they could not see the point at the time and declined.

Jahan had his cleft palate repaired but did not require cardiac surgery. His parents were told that they could access genetic counseling in the future, if they wished.

of which were autosomal trisomies, and the remainder involved the sex chromosomes. The most common chromosome abnormality affecting individuals that the health professional will encounter in practice is Down syndrome (trisomy 21), although there are many other possible chromosome abnormalities that can be identified.

Many hundreds of congenital abnormalities, involving all body systems have been described in the literature. For further detailed information see *Chapter 9* and the resources listed therein. The role of the genetic team is to try to determine whether the abnormality is isolated or part of a wider 'syndrome' or 'association', and to use the diagnostic information to guide management and provide a genetic risk assessment. At the very least this requires a detailed examination, and may require further diagnostic tests such as karyotyping.

8.4 Examination of the neonate

Diagnostic evaluation of a baby born with congenital abnormalities is the responsibility of a medical practitioner, but the nurse or midwife caring for the family needs to have an understanding of the components of the process in order to work with the family and to be able to initiate appropriate referral if necessary. Typical components of diagnostic evaluation include the following:

History	Examples of information gathered
Prenatal history	Any difficulties conceiving, use of folic acid supplements, maternal medical conditions
Perinatal history	Complications of pregnancy
	Details of screening results
	Labor history
	Type of delivery
	Baby's condition at birth and any resuscitation required
Family history	Previous liveborn children
	Previous miscarriages or stillbirths
	Three generation family tree
	Medical problems experienced by family members
	Details of any developmental problems or physical abnormalities in family members
	Congenital sensory abnormalities (hearing, vision) in family members
	Pregnancy losses in other family members

Physical examination	
Assessment of growth	Head circumference
	Length and weight of child (current and previous measurements since birth)
	Plot onto appropriate centile charts
General appearance	General impression of any pattern of features
Detailed examination	Systematic examination of the child's physical features
	Testing of reflexes, muscle tone and strength
	Listening to cardiac sounds

The history and examination will lead to an initial impression and differential diagnosis. This will guide subsequent diagnostic tests. A detailed examination checklist for an infant or child is shown in *Figure 8.3*.

8.5 Breaking bad news

It is important to realize that the way the family is told any possible diagnoses and how they are subsequently managed is only the first step in an ongoing

Measurements	Head and face	Eyes/ears	Limbs	Trunk	Skin
Length	Head shape	Eyebrows	Fingernails	Spine	Unusual skin patterns
Weight	Fontanelles	Eyelashes	Fingers	Chest shape	Birthmarks
Head circumference	Hair texture	Irides	Hand creases	Abdominal hernia	Skin tags
	Hair colour	Lenses	Size of hands	Genitalia	
	Hair quantity	Position of ears	Toenails	Testes	
	Mouth size	Size of ears	Toes		
	Mouth shape	Shape of ears	Hallux		
	Lips		Foot creases		
	Soft palate		Size of feet		
	Hard palate				
	Nose shape				
	Bridge of nose				
	Nares				
	Philtrum				
	Mid-face				
	Jaw				

Figure 8.3. Detailed examination checklist.

interaction with the medical profession. As with the breaking of any difficult news there are a number of issues to consider.

The environment. Ideally a quiet private environment should be provided. If requested by the family, other family members should be included.

The clinical encounter. The attitude of the health professional should be supportive, non-judgemental and take account of the cultural and ethnic values of the family. There should be respect for the autonomy of the family and, of course, for their confidentiality. It should be recognized that the family will go through a form of grieving and this needs to be taken into account.

Content. The medical facts as they are known should be given, which should include possible causes, the diagnosis and prognosis. Realistic prognoses if possible should be given, but include optimism if appropriate. The content should be tailored to the family's need to know and it should be emphasized that there will be further opportunities for discussion and clarification.

Extensive opportunities should be given for the family to ask questions and express their concerns. At all times the clinician should be honest and truthful about what they know and do not know. Information on patient support groups and other support services should be made accessible.

Knowing how and when to give information requires considerable skill on the part of the health professional. It should be recognized that immediately after the death of a child or the diagnosis of a serious problem, the parents might be unable to receive or understand complex information. Many individuals report that after hearing the initial news they 'shut down' and do not hear any ensuing information. For this reason it is very important to follow up with further conversations when the family are ready.

KEY PRACTICE POINT

Information about rare conditions may be based on studies that were done some time ago and prognoses may have changed due to advances in medicine and diagnosis. It is essential to get as much up-to-date information as possible before giving advice on the prognosis of any condition.

Parents may search for information in libraries or on the internet. Cases that are included in publications tend to be those that are at the more severe or unusual end of the spectrum, and parents should be warned about this and the fact that mild cases are frequently not diagnosed and therefore not reported.

CASE EXAMPLE   MARTIN FAMILY

A referral was made by telephone to the genetics department from the special care baby unit.

Baby Maria Martin had been delivered by Cesarean section. She was small for dates and had multiple abnormalities. The clinical geneticist visited the neonatal unit. The baby's father, David was there; her mother, Sally had not yet recovered sufficiently from the emergency Cesarean section to visit her baby yet.

The findings that were noted on examination were:

- bilateral cleft lip and palate
- microcephaly
- hypotonia
- highly arched eyebrows
- hypertelorism

The baby had already had a blood sample taken for karyotyping and an initial result was expected in 48 hours. An arrangement was made to see Sally and David together within the next few days.

The clinical findings suggested that Maria might have a condition called Wolf–Hirschhorn syndrome. However, the initial result of Maria's chromosome analysis was reported as normal. The geneticist also took a family history from David. Maria was their first baby and they had not had any other pregnancies. Wolf–Hirschhorn syndrome is caused by a deletion of the end of the short arm of chromosome 4. The geneticist therefore asked the cytogenetic laboratory to use a FISH probe to establish the presence or absence of a deletion (see *Section 4.4.1* for an explanation of FISH). The FISH test confirmed that Maria has indeed lost the end of the short arm of chromosome 4 as illustrated in *Figure 8.4*.

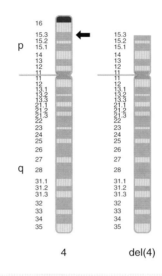

Figure 8.4. Ideogram showing a complete chromosome 4 and also 4p– (del(4)), as a result of an unbalanced translocation, typical of Wolf–Hirschhorn syndrome. Ideogram reproduced courtesy of the Cytogenetics Department, GSTS Pathology, Guy's Hospital, London, UK.

The cytogenetic analysis confirmed the diagnosis in Maria and showed that Maria had an unbalanced translocation. David and Sally were seen together and told about the diagnosis. Their first question was "How long will she live?". Older reports of children with this syndrome implied that many of them would die within the first 2 years of life. However, recent reports suggested that average survival might now be longer. This is probably because of improvements in medical treatments, but will also be the result of more diagnoses being made as cytogenetic techniques have improved.

Because Maria had been shown to have an unbalanced rearrangement, Sally and David also had their chromosomes checked. Sally was shown to have a balanced translocation involving chromosome numbers 4 and 6. This balanced translocation would have implications for the rest of the family and it was recommended that Sally tell her family and arrange for her parents to have their chromosomes checked. Sally said she could not do this; her parents, and particularly her mother, had been so distressed by what had happened that Sally felt they could not take on any more. They could not understand what had happened and wanted to blame somebody, and they also were full of guilt and worry about Sally. Sally felt that if her mother were shown to have the translocation she would not be able to come to terms with it and would blame herself. Sally and David wanted to concentrate on caring for Maria and looking after each other.

The birth of any baby born with an abnormality within a family will naturally affect all the members of that family. Grandparents in particular may find it difficult to know how best to help both their child and grandchild and, while being a source of support for the parents of the baby, may also feel excluded from the support and advice that is available for the parents. This is starting to be recognized by patient support groups who may offer specific advice and support to people in this situation. This can be brought sharply into focus when a diagnosis in a child has implications for the rest of the family. The health professional needs to be sensitive to these issues when caring for the family.

8.6 Genetic testing in the neonate

Increasingly detailed karyotyping in the neonate allows for more diagnoses to be made at an earlier stage. In the same way, the addition of molecular genetic techniques to careful clinical and pathological examination has increased the understanding of a diverse but individually rare group of neural, muscle and metabolic disorders that may present in the neonatal period. As before, an accurate diagnosis will allow specific information about prognosis and implications for other family members to be given.

Examples of conditions presenting in the neonatal period with muscle weakness include the following.

- Congenital myotonic dystrophy – autosomal dominant maternally transmitted.
- Type 1 spinal muscular atrophy (Werdnig Hoffman) – autosomal recessive.
- Centronuclear (myotubular) – X-linked myopathy.
- Mitochondrial myopathies – heterogeneous dominant recessive or mitochondrial.
- Prader–Willi syndrome – chromosomal.

The addition of molecular genetic techniques to the pathological and clinical examination may lead to diagnoses being made earlier than would otherwise have happened in the past. As discussed earlier in this chapter, the health professionals caring for the family need to ensure that any information given to the family is accurate and represents the current best knowledge.

CASE EXAMPLE	BABY AHMED

Baby Ahmed was born at term. He was a normal birth weight, but had very poor muscle tone and sucking reflex. He was not dysmorphic and had no relevant family history. The pediatrician examined him and considered the possible diagnoses. He considered asking for a neurological opinion and also asked for chromosomes to be checked. When the laboratory received the specimen they noted that hypotonia was mentioned on the referral card and ensured that the karyotype included a detailed examination of chromosome 15. A small deletion was detected at 15q11 in the Prader–Willi critical region. Blood samples were taken from the parents for chromosome analysis and their karyotypes were reported as normal. However, DNA probes were used to identify whether the deletion had arisen on the maternal or paternal chromosome. The analysis confirmed that the deletion was on the chromosome that had been inherited from the father. Prader–Willi syndrome is caused by the loss of the paternal contribution in a critical region of chromosome 15. This can happen through a variety of mechanisms: a deletion arising on the father's chromosome, inheritance of two copies of the father's chromosome 15 and none of the mothers, or by inheriting a gene that switches off that specific area on the father's chromosome 15 (for a more detailed discussion of imprinting see *Section 4.2.3*).

In Prader–Willi syndrome the usual history given is of a baby who is hypotonic at birth and then has feeding difficulties. However, at about the age of 2 years, the child will start gaining weight and will show an extreme interest in food. The weight gain is not only due to overeating; people with Prader–Willi syndrome seem to be lacking in the normal appetite control mechanisms and also have a lower metabolic rate with a high fat to muscle ratio. Children with the syndrome have mild to moderate learning difficulties and, although many of them start their education in mainstream school, they will normally need some educational help eventually.

As the genetic basis of diseases are clarified and more specific diagnostic and prognostic tests become available, the health professional will need accurate information and guidance to utilize this technology for the improvement of health care.

8.7 Neonatal screening

Screening is a process in which all individuals in a specific population are offered a test or asked a question to identify whether they have a higher than usual risk of that condition. The aim of any screening program is to do more good than harm and reduce the risks of morbidity associated with specific conditions. Neonatal screening started in most Western countries in the late 1960s with screening programs for phenylketonuria. Screening for congenital hypothyroidism was then added. Recently in the United Kingdom, universal neonatal screening for cystic fibrosis, sickle cell disease and MCADD (medium chain acyl-CoA dehydrogenase deficiency) has been adopted as policy. In some other countries screening for many more conditions is carried out, for example, the American College of Medical Genetics has recommended screening for a panel of 29 different conditions. However, this has raised concerns about the ethics of screening for many more conditions that may be untreatable and for which there is no evidence of benefit from early diagnosis[72].

8.7.1 Phenylketonuria

PKU is an autosomal recessively inherited inborn error of metabolism in which affected individuals are unable to metabolize the amino acid phenylalanine to tyrosine. This leads to high levels of phenylalanine that are neurotoxic. In the absence of treatment, nearly all affected individuals develop severe, irreversible learning difficulties together with neurological deterioration. These severe manifestations are now seen very rarely because of universal neonatal screening and subsequent dietary restriction. Classical PKU is caused by a deficiency of the enzyme phenylalanine hydroxylase (PAH); varying degrees of PAH deficiency, as well as disorders of other enzymes in the metabolic pathway (*Figure 8.5*), can all lead to high levels of phenylalanine. The disorder is therefore **heterogeneous**.

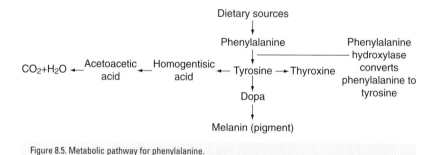

Figure 8.5. Metabolic pathway for phenylalanine.

All babies should have their phenylalanine levels measured on a dried blood spot (the **Guthrie test**). This should be done between 6 and 14 days after birth. Early diagnosis allows the initiation of a diet low in phenylalanine. In effect this means that protein intake is extremely restricted and supplementary amino acids are taken. Recent data suggest that this diet should continue at least until adulthood. There are special concerns about pregnancy in women affected with PKU and it is essential that low serum phenylalanine levels are maintained prior to conception and throughout the pregnancy (see *Section 7.2.3* for a discussion of the management of the pregnant woman with PKU). Although PKU is relatively rare (1 in 12 000 births), the fact that the prognosis is so devastating (if the problem is left untreated), that there is an effective treatment, and that a screening test with high sensitivity and specificity is available, make compelling arguments for universal **population screening**.

CASE EXAMPLE	KATY

Katy was just about to leave the postnatal ward after having her second baby when the midwife asked her to wait a few moments while they did the Guthrie test. Katy knew that all babies had a heel prick test just to check they were normal and was happy for this to be done. A week later she was contacted by a specialist nurse from the PKU service and was told that there was something wrong with the heel prick test and that her baby needed to be seen and the test repeated on a blood sample. Katy was given some information about PKU but was also told that it was possible that this first abnormal test result may mean nothing. She was given an appointment to see the pediatrician. The result of the second test confirmed the raised phenylalanine levels and PKU was diagnosed. When the pediatrician discussed PKU with Katy and told her that her baby was affected and would need to be on a special diet until he grew up, Katy was astonished. She had been given a leaflet about the heel prick test, but she had no idea of the implications of that routine test. The pediatrician also told her that the condition was genetic and that there was a one in four chance that any future children she had with the same father would also have the condition. She could not understand this as nobody in her family had this condition. The pediatrician explained that she and the baby's father each carried one copy of this faulty gene, but that by chance her son had inherited two copies and therefore could not make the enzyme necessary to convert phenylalanine to tyrosine. This meant that the levels of phenylalanine built up and would affect the way her son's brain developed. An appointment was made for her to see the rest of the team that cared for children with PKU, and the dietician went through the sort of diet her baby would need, including special formula milk. He would also need regular blood spot tests to check his levels of phenylalanine and to monitor his diet. Although Katy was reassured that treatment for her baby was possible, she was also worried about how she would manage preparing different foods for her two children, what she would do in the future about explaining the condition to her son, how he would cope as a teenager, whether she would be able to afford the special food he might need, and would she be able to do his blood spot tests?

8.7.2 Congenital hypothyroidism

Screening for congenital hypothyroidism is also performed on all neonates on the Guthrie blood spot. About 1 in 4000 babies are born with congenital hypothyroidism, 90% of whom will need lifelong treatment with thyroid

---

KEY PRACTICE POINT

Although information is given before population screening tests, a positive test result will still be unexpected. When giving positive screening test results, the practitioner should ensure they have enough information and are able to refer to the appropriate specialist service as soon as possible.

---

hormone replacement. A functioning thyroid is required for normal growth and brain development. As with PKU, if congenital hypothyroidism is diagnosed early enough treatment is effective. The condition can be caused by:

- ▪ failure of the thyroid gland to form normally – this is normally sporadic rather than genetic (80–85% of cases)
- ▪ an abnormality of the structure or function of the hypothalamus and / or pituitary – there are a variety of rare medical conditions associated with this central hypothyroidism, some of which are structural, some genetic (less than 5% of cases)
- ▪ an abnormality of the enzyme pathway necessary for thyroid hormone production or release – as with many inborn errors of metabolism, the majority of these are autosomal recessive genetic disorders (10–15% of cases)

8.7.3 Sickle cell disease, MCADD and cystic fibrosis

The practitioner should be aware of local policy in relation to newborn screening as the care pathways and implications for families may vary. In 2001, the UK government announced that universal neonatal screening for cystic fibrosis would be introduced together with screening for sickle cell disease. These programs are now developed and use the Guthrie blood spot samples. Sickle cell disease and cystic fibrosis have been discussed previously (*Section 7.2.4 and 7.2.5*). MCADD (medium chain acyl-CoA dehydrogenase deficiency) is a recessively inherited metabolic disorder. Deficiency of the enzyme means that there is a defect in the pathway that converts stored body fat to energy. Under conditions of fasting, toxic substances can build up which lead to serious neurological symptoms and even death. It is treatable by ensuring that the child does not go long periods without food and giving extra glucose during times of illness. Most children, if diagnosed and treated appropriately, have normal lives. There are a number of issues which caused concern when this expansion of the Newborn Screening Programme took place, for example:

- ▪ if DNA-based technology is used, carriers of these recessive genes will be detected as well as affected individuals – how should the parents of the baby be informed of their carrier status?

■ the hemoglobinopathies are more prevalent in specific ethnic minorities, so should screening be targeted to those ethnic minorities or be universal? The same issue applies to cystic fibrosis screening which is more prevalent among northern European populations.

There are also issues about the design and delivery of these screening programs. As discussed previously, practitioners caring for neonates should make themselves aware of policy in their area.

8.7.4 *Other neonatal screening programs*

The two national neonatal screening programs that have been in place the longest in the UK are for PKU and congenital hypothyroidism. Other screening programs for galactosemia, MCADD deficiency, and Duchenne muscular dystrophy are performed in other countries, or as pilots in specified regions within the UK.

8.8 Conclusion

Increased amounts of diagnostic and prognostic information will be made available through advances in genetics and this also requires the health professional to continue to gain the knowledge to apply these advances for the benefit of their patients. The issue of early diagnosis and the consequent uncertainty about prognosis has been discussed repeatedly in this chapter in relation to infancy. However, the increasing power of genetic advances to diagnose and predict is relevant at all stages of life as will be demonstrated in the chapters that follow.

> **Test yourself**
>
> **Q1.** When taking the family history from the parents of a newborn with a sub-mucous cleft palate, what might you specifically ask the parents about their own medical history and that of close relatives?
>
> **Q2.** The parents of a newborn boy who has been diagnosed with phenylketonuria are perplexed as to how he could have a genetic condition. They have not known of anyone else in the family with the condition and in fact had never heard of it before the screening test was done. How do you explain the lack of family history to them?
>
> **Q3.** Explain the difference between malformation and deformation. Give three examples of an abnormality caused by malformation and three caused by deformation.

Further resources

www.cafamily.org.uk/medicalinformation/conditions/azlistings/a.html — Contact a Family. *Information on rare congenital conditions.*

www.healthtalkonline.org/Pregnancy_children/Congenital_Heart_Disease — Health Talk Online – congenital heart defect. *True stories from parents of a child with a congenital heart defect.*

www.nlm.nih.gov/medlineplus/cleftlipandpalate.html and www.nlm.nih.gov/medlineplus/praderwillisyndrome.html – NIH Medline Plus. *Information on cleft lip and palate and on Prader–Willi syndrome.*

www.22q.org/ – The 22q11.2 Deletion Syndrome Foundation.

www.rarechromo.org/html/home.asp – Rare Chromosome Disorder Group.

Gorlin RJ, et al. (2001) *Syndromes of the Head and Neck.* Oxford: Oxford University Press. *Detailed text on dysmorphic syndromes.*

Jones KL (1997) *Smith's Recognizable Patterns of Human Malformation*, 5th Edition. Philadelphia: WB Saunders. *General text on dysmorphic syndromes with excellent description of formation of dysmorphic features.*

9 Childhood and adolescence

9.1 Introduction

This chapter is mainly concerned with those genetic conditions that become evident during childhood. In many cases, a genetic condition is first suspected when a child fails to reach their developmental milestones. As the health visitor or community practice nurse often has the closest contact with the family, and is responsible for monitoring the child's development, a number of referrals come from that source. However, if a child has a genetic syndrome, learning delay is rarely the only sign of the condition. A significant change in either the chromosome structure or a single gene will almost invariably also have some physical manifestations. These may be striking, such as a cleft lip, or very subtle, such as a double crown or small fingernails.

Physical characteristics that differ from the norm are termed 'dysmorphic features'. However, very few of us are made completely perfectly, and if you examine most children or adults you will find one or two mild dysmorphic features. In most families, there are significant physical characteristics that are the norm for those families, so it is always important to view a child in the context of their particular family.

> ### KEY PRACTICE POINT
>
> When talking to a family about the physical characteristics of a child, the family's view of the features is important. What may be unusual to the professional, may be 'just like Mum or Dad' to the family.

9.2 Why seek a diagnosis?

In some ways, finding the diagnosis may change very little when a child has health, educational or social problems due to a genetic condition. The genes are not changeable, and treatment is usually on a symptomatic basis. It could be argued that a child who has needs for therapy ought to have the therapy regardless of diagnosis. However, there are four key reasons for pursuing a genetic diagnosis.

The parent's need for information about the child. It has been demonstrated that parents who have a child with health or educational problems search for the reasons for those problems[73]. Without a diagnosis it is often difficult or impossible to have sufficient information about the likely prognosis, and questions about the child's future health or development cannot be answered. Some parents may even withdraw from a child emotionally, to protect themselves from further distress if they are unsure about the child's long-term survival.

Screening for complications. If a child has a genetic condition, they may be susceptible to complications or future health problems that could be avoided or treated promptly if the possibility of them occurring was known. For example, a child who has neurofibromatosis should have regular medical checks because they are susceptible to scoliosis and malignancy.

Facilitating access to support. While support for a child should be provided where there is need, in reality the diagnostic label often facilitates the parents in obtaining additional educational, social or financial support for their child.

Genetic risk assessment for other family members. Without a definite diagnosis in the affected child, it is difficult to assess the level of risk to other family members, including other current or future children of the parents. The parents may wish to have prenatal testing in a future pregnancy, and this would not be possible without diagnosis.

From a different perspective, having a diagnosis can lead to 'labeling' of the child. When a diagnostic label is given, the child may be judged according to reports of other children with the same condition, rather than on their own abilities. This may limit them in reaching their own potential, or more may be expected of them than they can achieve. If the term 'syndrome' is used in the diagnostic context, this may lead to misunderstanding outside the medical profession, as many people think only of Down syndrome when they hear the word syndrome.

CASE EXAMPLE   NATHAN

Nathan was the second child of Bob and Sue. Their first child, Helen, was a lively 7-year-old when Nathan arrived, and was doing very well at school. Nathan was a difficult child from the start – he wouldn't feed properly and never slept for more than 2 hours at a time. He seemed 'floppy' to his mother, in comparison to Helen. Nathan was very slow to smile, and didn't even try to roll over on his own until he was 8 months old. Sue and Bob were concerned, but other people reassured them that "boys are always slower than girls", and as he was quite a large baby he was bound to be "lazy". At 12 months, he was not able to sit unaided, and he was referred to the pediatrician by his health visitor. The pediatrician felt he was delayed, and did a series of tests, including a metabolic screen and chromosome analysis. No abnormalities were found on either.

By the time Nathan was 18 months, it was clear his development was severely delayed. He was still not able to sit properly without cushions. He was referred to the genetic service for further investigations, but as he had few dysmorphic features, finding a diagnosis was not possible at the time. Bob and Sue spoke to their health visitor about the agony of waiting for information about the cause of Nathan's problems. The uncertainty was making it harder for them to accept his condition, and also made it impossible for them to have information about his future development and prognosis. Sue said "It's like waiting, waiting, waiting every day, but I don't know what I'm waiting for, I'm just waiting. If I knew what we had to deal with, that would be easier, even if it was bad news, much easier to deal with that than the waiting."

9.3 Developmental delay

Developmental delay is defined as a delay in reaching the normal milestones within the normal age range for each milestone, for example, failure to walk before the age of 18 months. Development tasks are usually divided into categories, related to motor tasks, speech and cognition, and children may be delayed in their development globally (in all three areas) or specifically in just one category. For example, it is not uncommon to see children who are slower than normal in attaining speech, but who are progressing normally in other respects.

If delay is suspected, the child's development may be formally assessed using a recognized developmental test. This type of tool requires the child to complete a series of tasks, each designed to assess a different aspect of development, in the motor, speech or cognitive sphere. The tasks are assigned different point scores, and the number of points scored is compared with that expected for the child's age.

EXAMPLE OF DEVELOPMENTAL ASSESSMENT TOOL

To assess manipulative skills, the child is asked to build a tower of bricks, with points ranging from 1 to 4 for the number of bricks used.

In assessing vocalization, the child who used one word meaningfully would be allocated 1 point, while a child using several words with meaning would be allocated 4 points.

Locomotor skills involving the use of stairs would be judged, with a child who crawls upstairs attaining 1 point, and one who is able to run upstairs being allocated 6 points.

Parents will frequently have been the first to be concerned about the child, and may have raised their concerns previously. However, sometimes a parent will not have detected the delay, due to inexperience or avoidance, and so the news that the child is delayed may come as a shock. In a family where learning problems have been experienced by a number of family members, the child's situation may be considered to be the norm.

9.4 Learning disability

Children who have a learning disability are usually able to learn, but do so at a slower rate than their peers at the same age. This is important to explain to parents, who may feel their child will never develop the skills necessary for daily living. Learning disabilities can be defined further, as follows.

(i) Communication
- Expressive language disorder – difficulty using correct language.
- Articulation disorder – difficulty making speech sounds.
- Receptive language disorder – difficulty interpreting language.

(ii) Academic skills
- Dyslexia – difficulties reading the written word.
- Writing disorder – difficulties expressing through the written word.
- Arithmetic disorder – difficulties with number processes.

(iii) Motor skill disorders

(iv) Attention disorders
- Inability to focus attention is often accompanied by hyperactivity; the combination is termed Attention Deficit Hyperactivity Disorder (ADHD).

The reasons for learning disability are varied, and frequently there is no detectable genetic reason. However, the number of cases that appear to 'cluster' in families, and the genetic influences on brain development inevitably lead to the conclusion that there is a genetic influence in many cases of learning disability. It is often difficult though to make a firm genetic diagnosis unless the child also has significant dysmorphic features. Each child needs to be assessed formally and provided with educational support relevant to his/her own individual needs. Frequently the involvement of a community pediatrician or educational psychologist will be helpful.

9.5 What is dysmorphism?

Dysmorphism is defined as an unusual pattern of physical features. While there is a huge range of 'normality' in human characteristics, an abnormal gene or modified chromosome structure often alters the physical features in that child beyond the limits of the normal range. While these unusual characteristics are themselves usually completely benign, they provide clues as to the gene or chromosome abnormality in that child. Children who share the same genetic abnormality will share common characteristics and, although unrelated, may look very similar to one another. The most well known example of children who have the same chromosome abnormality looking similar is probably Down syndrome. Most people would be able to identify a person with Down syndrome because of the similar facial and body characteristics of those who have inherited an additional chromosome 21. Children with Down syndrome will also inherit some particular physical features that identify them as belonging to their family.

9.5.1 Common dysmorphic features

When a child with learning delay is referred to the genetic clinic for diagnosis, a thorough physical examination is essential, to detect any dysmorphic features that may give clues as to the diagnosis. A systematic examination (usually starting with the head and working down) is carried out so that small clues are not missed. To enable you to describe unusual features, it is helpful to become familiar with the anatomical terms used for different areas of the body, particularly the face (*Figure 9.1*).

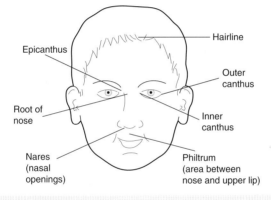

Figure 9.1. Facial landmarks.

Although there are hundreds of different dysmorphic features, some of the most common are as follows.

Head
- Microcephaly – head size below 3rd centile.
- Macrocephaly – head size above 97th centile.
- Hydrocephaly – head size increased due to excess fluid in ventricles.
- Delayed closure of fontanelles.
- Flat or prominent occiput.
- Craniosynostosis – abnormal joining of the bones of the skull, resulting in abnormal head shape.

Hair
- Abnormally thick or thin hair.
- Double crown.
- Widow's peak (see *Figure 9.2*).
- Sparse hair.

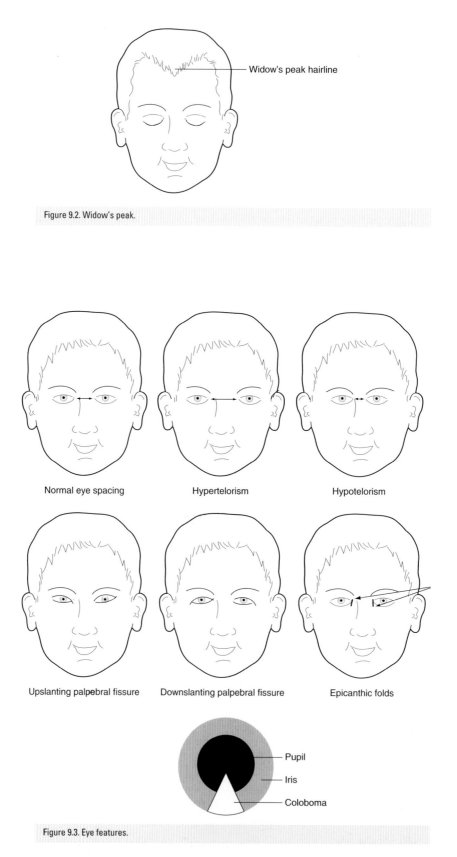

Figure 9.2. Widow's peak.

Normal eye spacing

Hypertelorism

Hypotelorism

Upslanting palpebral fissure

Downslanting palpebral fissure

Epicanthic folds

Pupil

Iris

Coloboma

Figure 9.3. Eye features.

Eyes

- Hypotelorism – short space between eyes (see *Figure 9.3*).
- Hypertelorism – long space between eyes.
- Slanting palpebral fissures (eye opening) – eyes either upslanting or downslanting.
- Epicanthic folds – folds of skin at inner canthus of the eye.
- Prominent eyes.
- Microphthalmia – small eye.
- Anophthalmia – absence of eye.
- Blue sclera.
- Coloboma – 'gap' in iris.
- Cataract.

Mouth

- Clefting of lips or palate – incomplete closure of lip or palate (see *Figure 9.4*).
- Prominent lips.
- Lip pits – small indentations in the skin.
- Macroglossia – large tongue.
- Hypoplasia of teeth enamel.
- Small or abnormally shaped teeth.
- Irregular placement of teeth.

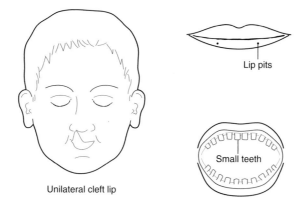

Lip pits

Small teeth

Unilateral cleft lip

Figure 9.4. Mouth features.

Ears

- Malformation of auricles.
- Low-set ears – upper edge of ear markedly lower than eye line (see *Figure 9.5*).
- Pre-auricular tags or pits – small skin tags or indentations anterior to the ear.

Hands/feet

- Brachydactyly – short fingers or toes.
- Clinodactyly – curvature of finger (usually 5th finger, see *Figure 9.6*).

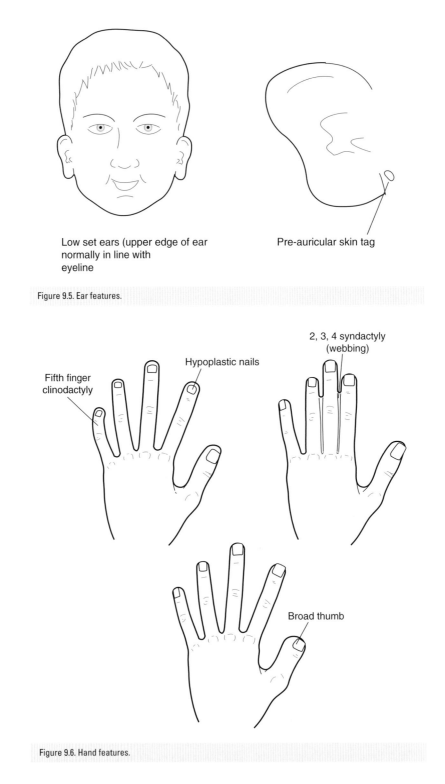

Low set ears (upper edge of ear normally in line with eyeline

Pre-auricular skin tag

Figure 9.5. Ear features.

Fifth finger clinodactyly

Hypoplastic nails

2, 3, 4 syndactyly (webbing)

Broad thumb

Figure 9.6. Hand features.

- Hypoplasia of thumb or fingers – digits less well developed than normal.
- Hypoplasia of metacarpals – metacarpal bones less well developed than usual.

- Polydactyly – additional fingers or toes.
- Syndactyly – webbing between fingers or toes.
- Broad thumb or toe.

Genitalia

- Hypospadias – abnormal site for urethral meatus, resulting in urethral opening on the shaft of the penis.
- Undescended testes.
- Unusually large or small penis/testes.
- Hypoplasia of labia majora – underdevelopment of the labia.
- Vaginal agenesis – absence of the vagina.
- Vaginal atresia – obstructed vaginal tract.

Stature

- Stature above 97th or below 3rd centile for age.
- Disproportion between trunk and limbs.

Skin

- Hyperhidrosis – excessive sweating.
- Hypohidrosis – decreased sweating.
- Altered skin pigmentation.
- Hemangioma – benign vascular tumor (strawberry-like).
- Thick or ichthyotic (scaly) skin.

Spine

- Neural tube defect.
- Scoliosis – lateral curvature of spine.
- Kyphosis – curvature of the spine resulting in 'bowing' of the back.

CNS

- Hypertonicity – high muscle tone.
- Hypotonicity – low muscle tone.
- Seizures.

Additional information may relate to 'internal' abnormalities, such as a heart defect, renal or ureteric anomalies, or tracheo-oesophageal fistulae. Further information on particular dysmorphic features can be found in any recognized textbook on dysmorphology or genetic syndromes.

It is very common for photographs to be taken of children in the clinic, to act as an aid to memory at a later stage. These form part of the child's medical records, and consent must always be sought from the parents (and child if old enough) before the photographs are taken.

Before and after a consultation, information about the child will be used to try and match the pattern of features in the child with those observed in other children. Increasingly this is done using computer software packages, such as the London Dysmorphology Database (see www.lmdatabases.com), or POSSUM. This type of software allows the principal features of the child to be listed, and a list of potential diagnoses that would be consistent with that pattern of features is produced. Of course, there is huge overlap in the patterns, so the skills of the geneticist are needed to differentiate the very probable from the less probable diagnoses. Inexperienced practitioners can look at a list of features and conclude that the child has a number of them and therefore a certain diagnosis must be correct. However, it is necessary to view the features as part of an overall appearance (or 'gestalt'), rather than as a number of unconnected features. The ability to assess a child in this way is attained with considerable clinical experience.

If the doctor seeing the child is unsure of the diagnosis, the case may be discussed in a wider forum to access a greater range of clinical expertise. This may take the form of a team meeting, a regional meeting or even a national meeting for the purpose.

Parents who are very eager to find a diagnosis in their child may latch onto reports of a syndrome in which the features appear to match their own child's. However, as has been said, there is a huge overlap of features, and the overall picture of the child is critical. For example, a child may present with a combination of features such as hypotonia, abnormal head circumference, developmental delay, and cleft lip or palate. There are a number of syndromes in which these features are seen, including the four described below, with vastly different causes and recurrence risks.

- Trisomy 13 – due to a chromosomal abnormality.
- Fetal valproate syndrome – due to the effects of the mother taking anti-convulsants during pregnancy.
- Crouzon syndrome – caused by a mutation in a single gene.
- Charge association – a combination of features often seen together but for which there is no single genetic basis known at present.

9.6 Genetic conditions in childhood

The conditions discussed here are chosen because they are commonly seen in a genetics clinic, because children with the conditions should be screened for complications, or because others in the family should be offered genetic counseling if the condition is diagnosed. More information on each condition can be obtained from the references listed at the end of the chapter or via the websites listed at www.scionpublishing.com/geneticsforthehealthsciences.

9.6.1 Cystic fibrosis

Cystic fibrosis (CF) is a recessive condition caused by a fault in the CFTR (cystic fibrosis transmembrane receptor) gene. This gene helps to control the flow of chloride ions through the cell membrane. As the balance of chloride ions across the membranes is abnormal, sodium and water balance is also affected. When a child inherits two faulty copies of this gene, the water/salt balance is altered in the mucus on the epithelial cells in the lungs and intestines. Recurrent respiratory infections occur due to the altered viscosity

Spencer Family

Luke Spencer is a 4 year old with moderate learning problems. Luke was late in reaching all his developmental milestones: he started walking at 19 months, and was regularly using just two words together until 30 months of age. Luke is similar to his father in coloring, with fair hair and blue eyes, but he is on the 97th centile for height, while his mother and father are both relatively short in stature. Tracy, his mother, is not overly concerned about Luke; her brother is 'slow' and she says with disarming honesty that the teachers thought she was very 'thick' at school. Luke goes to a local playgroup but has difficulty communicating with other children and spends a lot of time playing alone.

When bathing Luke one night, Tracy notices that his spine does not seem straight, and she rings the health visitor immediately. Luke is referred to a pediatrician, and is diagnosed with mild scoliosis. However, the pediatrician also notes Luke's learning delay and large head circumference, and takes a blood sample for chromosome analysis and fragile X testing.

Luke is found to have an expansion of the FRAXA gene, which has caused his learning delay and probably the scoliosis. Tracy is tested and found to be a carrier of the expansion. She feels vindicated at her lack of achievement at school, and feels that with a lot of support she can help Luke to achieve his potential. Having a firm diagnosis for Luke helps the family to argue for a place in the opportunity playgroup for Luke, and he has regular speech therapy.

of the mucus, and the child will not be able to digest food efficiently due to the effect on the pancreatic enzymes. A child with CF may have meconium ileus at birth, but recurrent chest infection, failure to thrive, and loose, smelly stools are the most common signs in infancy. Whilst a blood sample may be taken from the child for DNA analysis, the diagnosis of CF is still usually made on the basis of an abnormal sweat test. Treatment includes daily physiotherapy to remove secretions, the addition of pancreatic enzymes to the diet, and prophylactic antibiotics.

If a child has CF, both parents will be carriers of the condition, and each of their other children will have a one in four chance of inheriting the condition. If the gene mutations are known, prenatal diagnosis is possible in each pregnancy.

There are a large number of potential mutations in the CFTR gene, and clinical testing is usually only carried out for up to 32 of the most common mutations. Therefore, if a person has a CF carrier test that is negative, the chance that they are a carrier is greatly reduced, but there is still a small risk that they carry a rare mutation. The most common mutation found in Northern Europeans is the delta F508 mutation, so called because it involves a deletion at base number 508 in the CFTR gene.

Chester Family

Josie was three years old when her baby brother Samuel was born. Samuel had meconium ileus at birth, and was tested for cystic fibrosis at 6 weeks. His sweat test was abnormal, and cystic fibrosis was diagnosed. When speaking to the pediatrician, Josie's mother mentioned she had always been concerned about Josie's pale face and thinness, but had been reassured by her health visitor that some children are naturally pale and thin. A sweat test indicated that Josie also had cystic fibrosis. Blood samples were taken for DNA confirmation of the diagnosis, and both children had two copies of the delta F508 mutation in the CFTR gene.

9.6.2 Neurofibromatosis Type 1

Neurofibromatosis (NF) is an extremely variable condition, but due to the potential complications all children suspected of having NF should be referred to a pediatrician.

In many children, the appearance of multiple café au lait (CAL) patches on the skin will be the only sign. These benign coffee-colored marks usually appear between the ages of 1 and 5 years, and more than six CAL patches is diagnostic of NF. Children with the condition often also have a large head circumference and axillary freckling.

About 25% of children with NF have some type of learning difficulty, although this is often restricted to a particular area of learning, such as numeracy skills. Malignancies occur in a small percentage of children and for this reason unexplained signs and symptoms should be investigated promptly. As tumors can occur on the adrenal glands, blood pressure should be checked regularly. During adolescence and adulthood, those affected with NF usually develop some neurofibromata, which are small benign tumors of the nerve sheath. These can cause pressure on nerves, but mainly cause difficulty due to the visual appearance. Individual neurofibromata can be surgically removed.

The condition is dominantly inherited, and often one parent will have mild signs of the condition. However, new mutations occur in the gene, so a child may be the first in the family to have the condition. If a parent has the condition, each child will be at 50% risk of inheriting it.

9.6.3 Duchenne muscular dystrophy

As an X-linked condition, Duchenne muscular dystrophy (DMD) mainly affects males, though in very rare cases girls can be affected. The disease is caused by a mutation in the dystrophin gene on the X-chromosome, and may be carried by women who have no signs of muscular dystrophy.

This type of muscular dystrophy is generally diagnosed in boys when they are between 1 and 4 years of age. Generally the boy has been late in learning to walk, then is noted to have trouble climbing stairs or keeping up with his peers in terms of physical activity. The calves are usually large and firm. Greatly increased serum creatine kinase (CK) levels are a feature of the disease, and female carriers may also have raised CK levels. The diagnosis may be confirmed by DNA analysis or a muscle biopsy.

In the natural course of the disease, the large muscles are replaced by fatty tissue, and mobility is gradually reduced, with many boys requiring a wheelchair by the age of 12. Increasing deterioration of the heart muscle and restriction of breathing leads to death in the late teens or early twenties. A proportion of affected boys have learning problems.

When the diagnosis is made, the mother of the affected boy can be offered carrier testing. If a boy is the first member of the family to be diagnosed with DMD, his mother may be a carrier (2/3 of cases), or the mutation may have occurred for the first time in him (1/3 of cases). It is not always possible to identify the gene mutation in the affected boy. This can be a deletion, a missense mutation, or a nonsense mutation. If direct mutation testing for the mother is not possible, linkage analysis may be used to try to clarify her carrier risk, particularly if she has daughters (who may be carriers), or if she wishes to have more children. Prenatal diagnosis is possible if the mutation is known or if linked markers are available to differentiate between the X-chromosome with the mutation and the normal X-chromosome.

9.6.4 Phenylketonuria

A recessive condition, for which all newborn children in the United Kingdom are screened at 8 days of age (Guthrie test). Following a positive Guthrie test, a DNA test to confirm the presence of mutations in both copies of the phenylalanine hydroxylase (PAH) gene on chromosome 12 is performed. Children who are affected lack an enzyme needed to convert phenylalanine to tyrosine, hence the accumulation of phenylalanine in the body, and excretion of phenylketones in the urine. The increased phenylalanine levels damage the brain, and untreated children develop progressive severe mental retardation. Due to the lack of tyrosine, there is little pigment in the hair and skin.

Treatment with a low phenylalanine diet reduces the brain damage, and many children have normal intelligence. However, recent studies have shown that the diet needs to be continued beyond adolescence or regression can occur. Women with PKU who are at risk of becoming pregnant should be advised to adhere to the low phenylalanine diet as the increased levels in their blood can damage the brain of the fetus.

9.6.5 Albinism

Albinism (lack of pigment) can occur as a result of a number of different genetic conditions. Some children have ocular albinism, a form that affects mainly the pigment of the eyes. This can have no clinical manifestations at all but sometimes, as the eyes try to focus due to the lack of pigment, the child will develop nystagmus. Oculocutaneous albinism affects the hair, skin and eyes, and children with this form are at greatly increased risk of damage from the sun. Appropriate measures to protect their skin should be taken. In both forms of albinism, the child may benefit from dark glasses in sunlight. As albinism can be inherited in a dominant, X-linked or recessive form, assessment by a genetic counselor should be advised if the family are seeking information on recurrence risks.

9.6.6 Down syndrome

Children with Down syndrome have a number of characteristic physical features, including short stature, broad neck, flat facial profile, upslanting palpebral fissures, inner epicanthic folds, small hands and feet, and large protruding tongue. About 40% of babies with Down syndrome also have a congenital heart defect. During childhood they are likely to require additional help with schooling, with some attending mainstream school with assistance, and others attending special schools for children with learning difficulties. They may require surgical treatment that interferes with schooling, such as repair of hernias or congenital cardiac abnormalities. Eye surgery to 'normalize' the shape of the eyes is now being offered to some children, but remains controversial.

9.6.7 Turner syndrome

Girls with Turner syndrome are frequently diagnosed during childhood due to their small stature, or in adolescence because of the amenorrhoea. The syndrome is caused by the absence of the second sex chromosome; girls with Turner syndrome have just 45 chromosomes in all, including only one sex chromosome (45,X). This results in inadequate development of the ovaries, and most affected girls will not menstruate or ovulate. Infertility is therefore a feature of the condition. Some girls with Turner syndrome do have learning problems, although the majority are able to deal with normal schooling. Occasionally, a woman with Turner syndrome will have a child conceived using donor eggs. The syndrome usually occurs sporadically in a family and so the recurrence risk for the parents is therefore low.

9.6.8 Sickle cell disease

Sickle cell disease is a recessive condition, the signs and symptoms of which are due to the altered shape of the red blood cells. Abnormal changes in the structure of the hemoglobin molecules cause the cells to form a sickle shape. They are more fragile, and block small blood vessels, resulting in both pain and anemia.

A child who inherits two copies of the faulty gene is said to have sickle cell disease. An individual with one normal and one faulty copy of the gene is said to have sickle cell trait. The presence of one faulty copy is known to help protect the individual against malaria, hence the high proportion of the population in some areas of Africa with sickle cell trait. Sickle cell disease can be detected by a simple hemoglobin electrophoresis test.

Children with sickle cell disease are more prone to anemia, infection, delayed growth, and damage to kidneys or other internal organs due to blockage of blood vessels. In the neonatal period and early childhood they may be prescribed prophylactic antibiotics, and should be vaccinated against all childhood illnesses. Affected children should be encouraged to drink plenty of water, and folic acid may be given to reduce anemia. Carrier parents will have a one in four risk of having a child with the condition, in each pregnancy. Prenatal diagnosis is possible.

9.6.9 *Thalassemia*

Thalassemia is a recessive disorder causing an abnormality of hemoglobin molecules. As the condition results in severe anemia for the affected child, the current treatment consists of regular blood transfusions (about every 4–6 weeks). The excess iron in the body that is released when red blood cells are destroyed accumulates in the liver and heart, and the child also requires administration of an iron chelating agent (desferrioxamine) so that the excess iron can be excreted. Desferrioxamine is normally administered via a pump overnight. Some patients are now being successfully treated with a bone marrow transplant from a closely matched donor.

As there are two types of thalassemia, those affecting the alpha and beta hemoglobin chains, the exact diagnosis must be confirmed to enable the gene mutation to be found. If the mutation is not found, linkage studies can be used to track the faulty gene in the family, enabling prenatal diagnosis to be offered.

9.6.10 *The autistic spectrum / Asperger syndrome*

A number of children referred to the genetics clinic will have Asperger syndrome, or fit into the autistic spectrum of behavior. Asperger syndrome is classified under the *Diagnostic and Statistical Classification of Mental Disorders* (DSM-IV), and is defined as a condition in which there is little verbal or cognitive delay, but children with the condition have a marked lack of social skills and find it particularly difficult to interpret non-verbal communication. They are also prone to repetitive or obsessive patterns of behavior. Whilst there are a number of studies currently being conducted into the potential genetic cause of **autism**, other theories include the idea that autism is caused by an immunogenetic susceptibility to pathogens during pregnancy that affect a particular fetus but may not be harmful to others.

At present, if a child does not have significant dysmorphic features or other disabilities, it is unlikely that a genetic cause will be found to explain Asperger syndrome. Recurrence risks for the parents of a single child with Asperger syndrome are low and, as a specific gene mutation has not been identified, prenatal diagnosis is not possible.

9.6.11 *Fragile X syndrome*

Fragile X (FRAX) syndrome is the second most common cause of learning delay in boys (the most common is Down syndrome). The syndrome was named because of the fragile sites seen on the X-chromosome when the cells of an affected person were specially treated before culturing. It is an X-linked condition, and female members of the family may be carriers. Boys with the condition have moderate–serious learning problems and usually require special schooling. They are often tall in stature, and have large ears and testes. The syndrome is caused by an expansion in a particular gene on the X-chromosome, therefore a definitive diagnostic test is possible, and female members of the family can be tested for carrier status if they wish. Some females with the full expansion may also be affected and have significant learning difficulties.

9.6.12 *Hearing impairment*

Sensori-neural deafness is most often detected in children in infancy or early childhood. If both parents are hearing, then the condition is likely to be recessive, and future children born to the couple will have a one in four risk of hearing impairment. However, some forms of deafness are dominantly inherited. A careful family history is needed before recurrence risks can be given. Obviously, cases of conductive deafness due to infection, accidents or aging are not relevant to the genetic issues.

Some parents who have a hearing impairment themselves feel that the ability to communicate does not depend upon hearing, and do not therefore consider deafness to be a disability.

9.7 Genetic testing of children

Genetic testing of children has already been discussed in the first chapter, but it is relevant to revisit the topic here in more detail. Guidelines for testing children were suggested by the Clinical Genetics Society in 1994[74], based on studies performed at that time. However, there has been little empirical work to demonstrate whether individuals are actually harmed by testing in childhood for adult-onset diseases. As there is little evidence either way, it seems prudent to adopt the approach of doing least harm.

In general, if children are at risk of a condition that would require treatment or surveillance in childhood, then testing is justified. In some cases, testing a child to establish a diagnosis would not harm the child, and would possibly be of great benefit to the family. However, if a child is at risk of a condition that normally only affects adults, then testing is better delayed until the child can give informed consent. There is some evidence that when an individual is part of the decision-making process for testing, then they are better equipped to deal with the results of those tests. Testing children for carrier status would also fit into this category, as the results would only be of relevance to the individual when having children.

There are circumstances that arise in which withholding a test for a child may appear to damage the family unit; in those cases, consideration is given to the particular case, and expert advice is usually sought from other professionals in the field of genetics and related disciplines such as medical ethics. The establishment of clinical ethics teams in healthcare settings will be of great assistance in these cases.

9.7.1 Testing children – two case comparisons

Collins Family

Carol Collins is the mother of three children, Adam (11 years), Joe (8 years) and Amy (4 years). Carol has a family history of colon cancer, and had a colectomy at the age of 29 years, when she was found to have a bowel obstruction shortly after the birth of Amy. She found the diagnosis of colorectal cancer very difficult to come to terms with at first, but is now very positive about the surgery that "saved my life".

Carol was told that she had hundreds of polyps in her bowel, and that her children will need to be screened from the age of puberty.

She sees the genetic counselor, who explains the inheritance pattern (dominant) and offers to take a blood sample from Carol to see if the gene mutation for polyposis coli can be identified in the family. If the mutation is found, pre-symptomatic testing will be possible for the children. Carol is very keen, and a sample is taken. The counselor explains that it may be months or even years before the mutation is found. If the mutation is not found within a year, colonoscopy for Adam may have to be considered.

Four months later, the results arrive, the mutation has been found in Carol's sample, and she meets the counselor again to discuss testing for the children.

The counselor is aware that Carol very much hopes that the test will show that the children are 'all clear'. When the counselor asks her for her reasons for wanting the children tested, she says it is so she "doesn't have to worry about them any more". The counselor spends a lot of time encouraging her to consider the possibility of a positive result, that is, one that confirms the mutation is present in one, two or all of the children. One of the ways the counselor does this is to rehearse the news-giving session with Carol, using the terms that would be used for either outcome of testing. It is when the counselor rehearses saying "I'm sorry but Adam does have the gene mutation and will develop polyps in the bowel" that Carol starts to realize that the outcome of testing could go either way, and she breaks down. They talk about her guilt at possibly having passed the mutation on, and how desperately she wants to protect her children from worry and ill-health.

At the next session, the counselor and Carol talk about the children's readiness for testing. Carol feels she would like to know the status of all three children immediately. However, when they discuss how much understanding each of the children has about the situation, she agrees that only Adam would really understand the test and the reason for it.

At two further appointments, Adam and Carol are seen together, and blood is taken from Adam for a test, at his request. Four weeks later the counselor meets Adam and Carol to give them the news that Adam has inherited the gene mutation and colonoscopic screening is recommended. Adam has a colonoscopy 4 weeks later; several polyps are treated with laser therapy and Adam is scheduled for colonoscopy on an annual basis. The counselor arranges to meet Carol and Joe in 2 years to discuss testing for him.

Harding Family

Peter Harding is 42 years of age. He has inherited Huntington disease (HD) from his father Cyril. Peter and his wife Angie have separated, but still see a lot of each other. Angie helps Peter with his household chores, and has him to her place for a meal every second day, as he finds cooking for himself a bit of a problem, and he likes to spend time with their two children, Melissa and Jason. They all get along better since the divorce, as there aren't so many arguments now that Angie knows what is causing Peter's moods and she is able to deal with them better.

Angie is very anxious about Melissa and Jason. She knows they are at 50% risk and wants them to be tested. When she meets the genetic counselor to discuss testing, she says that she is worried Melissa might get pregnant, but if she knows the baby is at risk of HD that might make her more careful.

The counselor explains that many people at risk of HD do not want to know their status, preferring instead to live with the risk. She also explains that informed consent is needed for such a test, and that children under 18 years are not tested except in exceptional circumstances.

Angie brings Melissa to the next appointment, and it is clear that Melissa does not want to be tested at present. She is very upset about her father's illness, and is trying to put her own risk out of her mind and "just get on with life". Angie asks the counselor to take a sample from Jason without telling him what it is for, because he is a worrier. Again, the counselor explains that testing without informed consent is not ethical.

The genetic counselor offers Angie several further appointments to discuss her own anxieties for her children. She leaves the door open for Angie to contact her again if she wants further counseling, and tells the children they can see her again to discuss their risks in the future if they wish.

9.8 Genetics of common complex disorders and traits affecting children

The understanding of the genetic influences on complex disorders is expanding at a great rate. Previous discussion in this chapter has focussed on classically inherited disorders caused by single genes. Even these disorders are known to be more complex than previously thought. For example, it is now known that carriers of a pre-mutation or small expansion in the fragile X gene can have effects from it. Women may have early ovarian failure and have an early menopause, whereas males may develop an ataxia at an older age; these have significant implications for counseling in these families[75].

Spencer Family

Luke is now 9 years old and his mother Tracy is planning another baby. She feels that after their early problems with Luke he is now more settled and the time is now right for her and her partner. She is in regular touch with the fragile X support group and has heard about a new technique called PGD which means that she would not have to have prenatal diagnosis and end a pregnancy if it was affected. She has also heard that some women who carry what she calls a small fragile X gene, may go through an early menopause. She was devastated when she found that although she was only 34, her hormone profile showed that there would be very little chance of her becoming pregnant and the PGD team recommended that she did not go through IVF treatment.

Although there are regular research reports saying that new genes have been discovered for various conditions, in reality these findings have little direct implication at the moment for patient care. To illustrate some of the complexity, two examples will be discussed briefly: asthma and obesity.

9.8.1 Asthma

It has been known for some time that asthma and asthma-related traits such as wheezing and atopic dermatitis run in families. Some genetic studies have focused on finding associations between genetic variants in biological pathways that were already thought to be associated with asthma. A number of susceptibility genes have been identified in pathways associated with innate immunity and immunoregulation: in genes associated with T cell differentiation, in genes associated with the biology of the epithelium, and in genes associated with lung function. Other genes have also been identified using traditional linkage approaches in families. More recently, a large genome-wide association study has identified a new gene of unknown function that appears to be significantly associated with susceptibility to asthma. What this gene may do and how it contributes is not known. It is clear that the end phenotype of asthma is a complex interaction between the various genetic and environmental factors. In addition, it seems that most of the factors that affect the start and progression of allergic inflammation also have to act within a particular developmental window, i.e. within a narrow window of time in early life. The research is leading to greater understanding of the relevant mechanisms that may be important, but as yet it is too early for the development of effective prevention or treatment strategies[76].

9.8.2 *Obesity*

Obesity is a serious public health concern in many countries and there has been particular focus on obesity in children. Rising levels of obesity are predicted to lead to a huge surge in associated diseases such as metabolic syndrome, type 2 diabetes, and cardiovascular disease. The environmental causes of obesity are relatively straightforward, namely excess dietary energy intake and too little physical activity, but the genetic factors are more complex. There are rare single gene disorders where obesity is a symptom, but genes underpinning these disorders do not seem to be associated with obesity in the general population.

Genome-wide association studies have demonstrated association between relatively common genetic variants and obesity. A recent meta-analysis of 15 previously published genome-wide association studies, with a combined total of more than 32 000 individuals, looked for genetic variants associated with BMI[77]. This meta-analysis confirmed previous findings and noted that a number of the genes identified are involved in the central nervous system, which may indicate the importance of neural control of weight regulation. Further support for the role of behavioral aspects in the control of weight comes from a study investigating a known obesity-associated gene, FTO. Children with the high risk allele were more likely to choose high energy food than children with the low risk allele, although they did not consume more food. The high risk allele was associated with greater energy consumption and greater fat rather than muscle mass. There was no association with metabolic rate, leading the authors to suggest that the gene may have a role in food preference rather than control of appetite or metabolism[78].

As these two examples show, while the scientific discoveries from genetic studies are leading to increased knowledge, the opportunities for therapy and treatment are no closer. Environmental interventions, particularly in the case of obesity, are likely to be the most effective. The old advice of eating healthily and taking more exercise still holds true, regardless of the genetic discoveries.

9.9 Genetic healthcare issues in adolescence

9.9.1 Transfer of care from pediatric to adult services

A young person who is affected with a genetic condition such as cystic fibrosis or muscular dystrophy will have healthcare provision under the pediatric services until at least the age of 16 years. In reality, healthcare for these clients usually continues to be provided by a pediatrician beyond that age, partly because of the long-term relationship that has been built up with the young person and their carers. However, sometimes this occurs because adult services for these clients are not as well developed as pediatric services. This is in part due to the changing survival rate; adult services for such clients were not in demand when most children died from the condition. In other situations, children are discharged from pediatric care but there is a noticeable gap in healthcare for them in adult services.

A new group of patients with genetic diseases that are now receiving treatment are those with lysosomal storage diseases. The lysosomal storage diseases include disorders such as Gaucher disease, Fabry disease, Pompe disease, and the mucopolysaccharidoses. Enzyme replacement therapy (which is a lifelong therapy), normally given by infusion, is not a cure but, depending on the disorder, it has been shown to stop the development of some of the complications and also extend life expectancy[79]. Some of these conditions can manifest in adults and others in children. As individuals live longer with these conditions and some aspects of the diseases are treated, new disease complications will emerge. The survival of children who now require long-term treatment for chronic conditions will challenge the provision of healthcare services.

Those caring for young people should, however, bear in mind their emotional and psychological needs as well as the physical needs; it may not be very positive for a young person of 19 or 20 to be cared for in a pediatric clinic. Adolescence is normally a period in which young people establish their independence, gradually loosening the ties to their parents. Disability brings with it additional dependence on others and this is reinforced by having to use pediatric facilities.

In some areas, a joint pediatric/adult clinic is set up to expedite the effective transfer of care, and if this can be organized it may be very helpful in ensuring the young person's physical and psychological needs are met.

9.9.2 Issues of sexuality and reproduction

Experience working with disabled teenagers has shown that they think about their own sexuality and reproductive issues far earlier than their parents realize! Evidence suggests that young people often avoid talking about such issues with their parents to protect them, but that these issues are very important to them. It is therefore helpful to be able to offer young people affected with a genetic condition opportunities to talk freely about their condition and ask questions. A school nurse, practice nurse, family doctor or genetic counselor can offer this, but sometimes it is possible to set up contacts between special schools and genetic counselors, so students can be offered the chance to speak privately to the counselor.

Although young people may ask about the chances of their own children developing the same condition, they are frequently concerned about their own future prognosis, and wish to speak with someone who has experience of the condition.

9.9.3 Informing the adolescent about genetic risk

One question that is often asked by parents who have children at risk of a genetic disease is "When should I tell my child about the risk?". Parents frequently feel the conflict between believing a child has the right to know about the risk, and wishing to protect the child from worry.

Studies show that those who are at risk wish to be told, mainly so that they have the opportunity to make life choices, taking the risk into account. There is no 'right time' to tell a child, but it appears that individuals who grow up knowing about the condition in the family are able to adjust and live with the risk more easily than those who are told in adulthood. Those at risk find it especially hard to adjust if others in the family knew of the condition, and withheld the information from them. This secrecy that exists in many families at risk of a genetic condition creates anger and distrust and, hard as it is for parents, it seems much more positive to tell children of their risk and so empower them to consider the options available and make their own decisions.

A study focusing on telling adolescents about their risk of polyposis coli showed that it was better to avoid telling the child in the period of early adolescence. Children who were told either before 10 years or after 13 years were able to accept the news more easily than those who learnt of their status during the critical period between those ages. As so much change occurs at that time, when the child is struggling to develop a sense of their independent self, this is not surprising.

CASE EXAMPLE   **JUDITH**

Judith was the eldest of three children born to Harry and Helen. Harry's father died of pre-senile dementia at 48 years of age. At that time the family were unaware that this could be an inherited condition. Harry's much older sister developed the condition in her 40s, and it was then that the family began to suspect it could be familial. However, Helen and Harry both wanted children, so went ahead with their family plans.

Harry was diagnosed when Judith was 17 years of age. Her brother was 15 and her younger sister 14 years of age. Judith suspected the condition was familial, but her mother denied this vehemently. Finally Judith sought medical advice prior to her marriage. She found out that her father's condition was an inherited form of pre-senile dementia and that she was at 50% risk of developing it herself. She was furious at having been lied to, and an argument with her mother followed. Judith's mother's rationale for not telling her children was that she didn't want them to be made unhappy.

Judith felt her brother and sister should also be aware of their risk. She told her brother, and her mother warned her that if she told the sister she would be cut off from the rest of her family. As Judith was very concerned about her father she wanted to avoid this. She felt forced to comply.

Subsequently, and without the knowledge of the family, Judith's young sister found out about her risk, and when she became pregnant had a termination because of her worry about the condition. She went through this completely unsupported by the family because she felt unable to share her knowledge with anyone.

9.9.4 Loss of a parent in adolescence

In a genetics clinic there will be a considerable proportion of clients who have lost a parent during their childhood or adolescence. This is especially true of clients seeking advice about a family history of cancer, and this history may have a strong influence on decision-making. For example, a woman who was in her teens when she lost her own mother due to breast cancer will have been influenced by that event. Her attitude to her own health, her body, her sexuality and her relationships will have been affected, and this may alter radically her approach to genetic testing, screening programs, breast self-examination and prophylactic surgery. In particular, women who lost a parent before they were independent frequently express a need "not to leave my children without a mother", and this may influence them to opt for radical prophylactic surgery.

9.10 Conclusion

In childhood and adolescence, genetic conditions may cause a range of physical and/or learning problems. These will have an impact on the child's social and educational development, and healthcare services for these children must address these areas as well as the treatment or prevention of illness. As the child grows into adolescence they may face particular difficulties in establishing independence, and sensitivity is needed to enable the young person to create independence at an appropriate level.

Test yourself

Q1. Joe is 18 years old, and has learning problems. He attends a special school, and prefers to play with children who are about 3 or 4 years younger than himself. His reading age is 9 years.

The cause of Joe's problems has not been investigated. It is suspected that he may have fragile X. His sister Marie is married and worried that she may have a child with learning problems.

A blood sample from Joe could be tested for fragile X and chromosome abnormalities. The results of these tests would help the counselor advise Marie about the risks of her children having learning problems. Joe is reluctant to give a blood sample as he hates needles. What are the rights of Marie and Joe in this instance? Should Joe be persuaded or even coerced into giving a sample? Do Marie's future children have any rights in this matter?

Discuss with colleagues what you would do if (a) Joe was your patient, (b) Marie was your patient. Is there an ethical solution? Would your response change if Joe was 10 years old?

Q2. How would you record the following features in the medical records, using the accepted terms?

a) Widely spaced eyes.
b) Shorter than usual distance between the nose and upper lip.
c) Additional finger on the right hand.
d) Webbing between the 2nd and 3rd fingers on both hands.

Q3. What do the following terms mean?

a) Hypotelorism.
b) Brachydactyly.
c) Macroglossia.

Further resources

www.cafamily.org.uk/medicalinformation/conditions/azlistings/a.html — Contact a Family. *Information on rare congenital conditions.*

www.ncbi.nlm.nih.gov/sites/entrez?db=omim — Online Mendelian Inheritance in Man. *Resource on genetics, natural history and testing of all genetic diseases.*

Borry P, Stultiens L, Nys H, Cassiman JJ, Dierickx K (2006) Presymptomatic and predictive genetic testing in minors: a systematic review of guidelines and position papers. *Clin Genet.* **70**: 374–81.

Clarke AJ (1998) *Genetic Testing of Children.* Oxford: Bios Scientific Publications. *All aspects of genetic testing debate covered in detail.*

Jones KL (1997) *Smith's Recognizable Patterns of Human Malformation,* 5th Edition. Philadelphia: WB Saunders. *Seminal text on dysmorphic syndromes.*

Adulthood

10.1 Introduction

This chapter is concerned mainly with those conditions that have an effect on the health of a person during their adult life. These are usually termed the adult-onset conditions but, due to the variability of some conditions, there may be a huge range in the age of onset, and even within the same family the onset of signs and symptoms may occur at vastly different ages. While there are many adult-onset conditions, for simplicity in this chapter we will focus mainly on four groups of conditions: familial cancers, neuromuscular disorders, psychiatric disorders, and genetic hemochromatosis.

10.2 Familial cancer

10.2.1 *Genetic basis of cancer*

Due to the high incidence of cancer in the population, there will be some history of cancer in virtually every family. However, in the majority of cases, cancer occurs as a sporadic event as a result of changes in the genes in a particular cell (somatic change). Due to the increased public awareness of familial aspects of cancer, there has been a sharp increase in the number of people enquiring about their own risks and the steps they might be able to take to reduce their chance of developing cancer and/or to detect tumors at an early stage, to increase their chances of survival. Although there are a number of rare cancer syndromes, such as von Hippel–Lindau disease, in general the majority of familial cancer referrals will be connected with colorectal cancer or breast/ovarian cancer. If a person presents with a family history of cancer, we need to try to work out if a number of cancers have occurred co-incidentally in the family, or if there is a family gene being inherited by some family members.

The function of some genes is to help prevent the growth of tumors or cancers; these are called tumor suppressor genes. Whenever new cells are produced in the body to replace dead or damaged cells, the tumor suppressor genes limit the number of new cells, thus preventing overgrowth of the tissue. If the particular sequence of these genes is correct, then the protective action of the genes is intact. However, the genetic material is copied over and over again during the person's lifetime as new cells are made. Each time the gene is copied there is the potential for a mistake to be made in the sequence of base pairs. If one copy of the gene becomes faulty or is 'spelt incorrectly', then the remaining normal copy will usually still protect against cancer. However, if both copies of that particular gene become faulty then the protection against cancer will be removed, and the person has a much higher chance than previously of developing a tumor.

Knudson[80] first described the two-hit hypothesis in development of cancer in retinoblastoma, and the hypothesis helps us to make sense of what occurs in familial cancer. If a person is born with one faulty copy of a gene, then they are likely to develop cancer at a younger age, because they only need one more accidental fault in the gene to occur to make both copies faulty (*Figure 10.1*). If

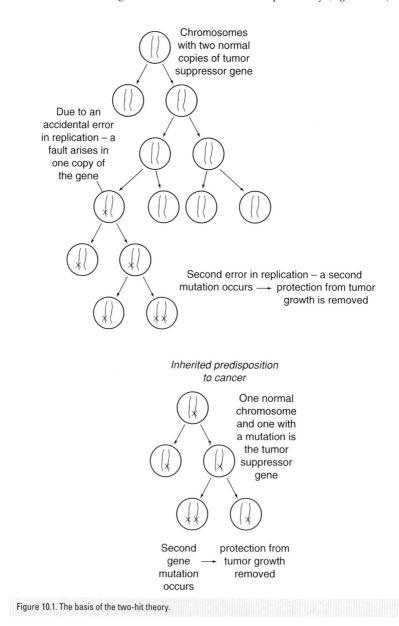

Figure 10.1. The basis of the two-hit theory.

you are interested in knowing more about this theory, see Chial (2008) in *Further resources*.

When we look at a family history, there are three main indicators that a gene mutation may be causing a predisposition to cancer in the family.

- Are the cancers in the same or related parts of the body?
- Is there cancer in more than one generation of the family?
- Have people in the family developed cancer at a younger age than you would generally expect?

Take, for example, the cases of two women referred with a family history of breast cancer, Gail and Helen.

In both cases, the referral letter gave the same information:

> *Dear counselor*
> *This woman is 38 years of age. Her mother had breast cancer, and her grandmother also died of cancer.*
> *She is very worried about her own risk. Can you assess and give me some guidance about screening for her?*
> *GP*

The counselor sees both women, and takes a family history.

Gail. In Gail's case, her mother had breast cancer diagnosed when she was 63 years old. The grandmother who died had cancer of the bladder at 72 years of age (*Figure 10.2*). Gail is at low risk because although there are two generations affected with cancer, cancer of the bladder is not known to be caused by the same gene mutation as cancer of the breast, and both cases occurred in older age, making them more likely to be due to the aging process rather than an inherited genetic predisposition. Additional screening for Gail is not indicated.

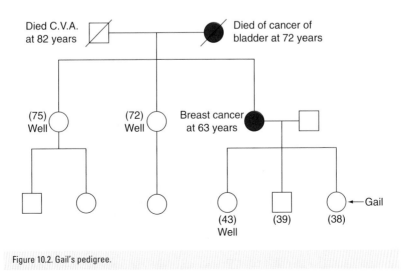

Figure 10.2. Gail's pedigree.

Helen. Helen's mother was diagnosed with breast cancer at the age of 38 years (*Figure 10.3*). Although the treatment at the time was thought to be successful, she subsequently died after developing metastases 3 years later. Helen was only 15 years old at the time of her mother's death. Helen's maternal grandmother, Hilda, had 'stomach' cancer at 58 years and died within two weeks of diagnosis. A check with the cancer registry showed that this was in fact ovarian cancer. Breast and ovarian cancer are known to be caused by the same gene mutation, Helen's mother was very young when the cancer was diagnosed, and there are two successive generations affected. It is therefore likely that in this family there is a gene mutation that increases susceptibility to breast and ovarian cancer. Helen is at high risk, and should be offered both breast and ovarian cancer screening.

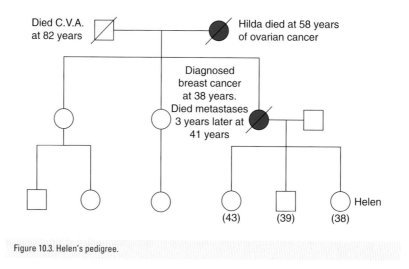

Figure 10.3. Helen's pedigree.

10.2.2 *Breast and ovarian cancer*

Guidelines for referral to the genetic service. Health professionals working in primary or secondary care will often be faced with a client who has questions about their own family history of cancer. It is helpful to have some guidelines as to whether a history is likely to be significant.

For practical purposes, it is useful to determine the level of increased risk, as this may provide an indication of the type of referral and screening/management options that would be appropriate for a particular individual. If a person is assessed as having 'similar to population' risk (lifetime risk of less than 17%), no additional referral or screening is indicated. If the person has an increased risk (lifetime risk of 17–30%), then referral to a secondary center for assessment and screening is indicated. People assessed as being at high risk (greater than 30% lifetime risk) should be referred to the genetics specialist team so that genetic testing can be considered and the implications for the wider family addressed (*see* Lalloo *et al.* in the *Further resources* section).

Breast or breast/ovarian cancer history indicating increased risk (17–30% lifetime risk):
- One 1st degree relative and one 2nd degree relative from the same side of the family diagnosed after average age of 50 years.

  or
- Two 1st degree relatives from the same side of the family with an average age of diagnosis over 50 years.

  or
- One 1st degree relative diagnosed before the age of 40 years.

Breast or breast/ovarian cancer history indicating possible high risk (greater than 30% lifetime risk):
- Three close relatives (1st or 2nd degree) from the same side of the family diagnosed at any age.

  or
- Two 1st degree relatives from the same side of the family with an average age of diagnosis under 50 years.

  or
- One 1st degree and one 2nd degree relative diagnosed before the average age of 50 years.

  or
- One male 1st degree relative (father or brother) with breast cancer diagnosed at any age.

  or
- One 1st degree relative with bilateral breast cancer, with the first cancer diagnosed under 50 years.

Breast and ovarian cancer:
- One 1st or 2nd degree relative diagnosed with ovarian cancer at any age.

  and
- One 1st or 2nd degree relative with breast cancer at any age, from same side of the family (one should be a 1st degree relative).

NB *A 1st degree relative means a parent, brother, sister, or child. A 2nd degree relative is a grand-parent, aunt, uncle, nephew, niece or grandchild.*

Many families are not aware that inherited forms of breast and ovarian cancer can also be passed down through the father's side of the family, therefore the family history from both sides of the family could be significant. Men can carry the faulty gene, but of course are less likely to develop this type of cancer since they have no ovarian and very little breast tissue. Women who are of Ashkenazi Jewish origin are at higher risk, due to the presence of particular gene mutations in that population, and should be assessed even if the history does not meet the criteria stated above. In addition, if the individual has a history of unusual tumors such as gliomas or sarcomas, advice should be sought from a genetic specialist as the pattern of cancers may be due to a fault in a gene required for DNA repair.

Tables developed by researchers such as Claus *et al.*[81] can be used to determine the level of risk to each person in the family, and as a guideline for screening recommendations. Software packages such as *Cyrillic* are based on these tables and can also be used for this purpose. However, a level of expertise and underlying knowledge is necessary in order to interpret the family history data correctly and so use the tables accurately. The guidelines published by the National Institute for Health and Clinical Excellence (NICE) are a valuable resource, indicating levels of risk and appropriate screening[82].

Screening protocols. At present, there are no ideal methods for screening women for breast cancer. Women are advised to examine their own breasts after a period each month, and to seek medical advice if they see or feel changes in the breast or armpit. Mammography is used extensively, but is less sensitive in pre-menopausal women than in those who are post-menopausal, and so is less effective in the high-risk group for whom additional screening is needed. Practitioners working in the UK will find that the screening programs offered to women conform to the guidelines issued by NICE. These state that women whose risk of developing breast cancer is above the population risk should be offered annual mammographic screening between the ages of 40 and 49 years. Women who have a known genetic mutation are now offered MRI screening from 30 to 49 years, while those known to have a TP53 mutation are offered MRI screening from 20 years of age.

Similarly, ovarian screening is not highly sensitive. Ultrasound of the ovaries is used, but may not detect a tumor. The CA125 test, which is a measurement of a hormone excreted when there is a malignancy in the ovary, may also be used. If there is a suspicion of a tumor on ultrasound or CA125 testing, an ovarian biopsy will be performed. Vaginal examination may detect enlargement of the ovaries. Screening does detect some ovarian cancers, but US studies have shown that it may also result in unnecessary surgery for some women[83]. It is not clear whether screening actually has an impact on the mortality rates for ovarian cancer, but clinical trials are in progress.

Levy Family

The genetics team received a copy of a referral letter sent to the breast surgeon. Mrs Becky Levy was a woman of 30 years of age who was concerned about a lump in her breast. She had a fast-track appointment to the breast clinic and a benign cyst was found in her left breast. She was then asked to attend an appointment with Gillian, the genetic nurse, to discuss her family history.

Becky was the youngest of three sisters. She also had two older brothers. Her maternal grandparents had emigrated from Eastern Europe but both were deceased and there was little family knowledge of their backgrounds. Becky said the family preferred 'not to think about the past'. Her paternal grandparents were also deceased; there was even less information about them as Becky's father had been raised by a cousin because of the early death of his own mother from cancer.

Becky was able to tell the genetic nurse that her eldest sister had breast cancer at the age of 49 years. Her other sister and her brothers were all well. Her father (aged 77 years) had severe coronary artery disease and her mother (74 years) was well except for having to cope with Type 2 diabetes that had been diagnosed 10 years earlier.

On the face of it, Becky's family history of breast cancer was not greatly significant. Her sister had been diagnosed at 49 years and her paternal grandmother had cancer, the site of which was unknown. However, Becky's family were of Ashkenazi Jewish origin, and therefore Gillian was aware that they may well have had one of the inherited mutations known to be passed down in Ashkenazi families. The lack of family history due to migration also meant that there could have been other cases further back or in the wider family. Gillian therefore discussed the possibility of genetic testing with Becky. Becky agreed to talk to her eldest sister, Ruth, and ask her to attend the next appointment. Because Ruth had already had breast cancer, it was likely that if there was a genetic mutation in the family, Ruth would have inherited it. Although in Ruth the test was not a pre-symptomatic one, full consent and preparation for the result was important. Subsequently Ruth was tested and found to have a BRCA1 mutation. Becky chose to have pre-symptomatic testing and had not inherited the familial mutation, although her other sister chose not to be tested.

While Gillian was pleased that Becky was so relieved, she also emphasized that Becky could, like all other women in the general population, still develop breast cancer in the future and she should attend for routine breast cancer screening when this was offered.

Lifestyle advice for women at increased or high risk of breast cancer.

- Women should be advised not to smoke and to limit their alcohol intake to the recommended levels.
- Women who are overweight should be advised that this could contribute to a higher risk of breast cancer.
- Those women who have a baby should be advised that breastfeeding reduces the risk of breast cancer.
- Women should be advised about the use of HRT, taking into account the family history and the indications for HRT use. If women with an increased risk of breast cancer use HRT, this should be for the shortest period of time and using as low a dose as possible.
- Women who are 35 years or older and who have an increased or high risk of breast cancer should be made aware that use of oral contraception may increase that risk. However, it has been shown that women with a *BRCA1* mutation may actually have a reduced risk of ovarian cancer associated with oral contraceptive use, and should have the opportunity to discuss the potential risks and benefits with a specialist.

10.2.3 *Colorectal cancer*

When there is a history of colorectal cancer, we can categorize families into two levels of genetic risk, according to the amount of evidence supporting the presence of a gene mutation in the family. The first group of families are those where it appears very likely there is a dominant gene involved.

Familial adenomatous polyposis. Also called polyposis coli, FAP is due to a change in the *APC* gene, and results in multiple polyps growing inside the colon. These predispose to adenocarcinoma of the colon or rectum. If a person has the gene mutation, they are almost certain to develop dozens or even hundreds of polyps in their teens or 20s. Family members who are at risk should be screened annually by colonoscopy, from the age of about 12 years. If a person develops multiple polyps, colectomy is performed to reduce the cancer risk, often in the late teens. This is an autosomal dominant condition and therefore every child of an affected person has a 50% chance of inheriting the condition.

Hereditary non-polyposis colon cancer. If there is a strong family history of bowel cancer, but the affected individuals have not had multiple polyps, then one of the genes known to cause hereditary non-polyposis colon cancer (HNPCC) is suspected[84]. In addition to colorectal cancer, these gene mutations may also be implicated in endometrial, stomach, ovarian and urinary tract cancer.

The genes involved are **mismatch repair genes** (such as *MLH2* and *MSH2*), which have a role in repairing faults in the DNA sequence. The mismatch results in microsatellite instability, so a tumor sample can initially be tested for instability to try and locate the site of the gene mutation. Regular screening by colonoscopy from about 25 years of age is recommended if a person is at risk of HNPCC.

Colorectal cancer pre-disposition. There are a number of families where there is *some* evidence for the presence of a gene mutation, but the cancers in the family may also have occurred sporadically. In these families, screening may be undertaken on a less frequent basis, for example, 5 yearly, starting 5 years before the mean age of diagnosis of colorectal cancer in that family.

Lovett[85] developed some guidelines that help to clarify the risk when there is a family history of colorectal cancer (without multiple polyps):

Family history	Lifetime risk
More than two 1st degree relatives affected	1 in 3
Two 1st degree relatives affected	1 in 6
One 1st degree relative < 45 years affected	1 in 10
One 1st degree relative and one 2nd degree relative affected	1 in 12
One 1st first degree relative > 45 years affected	1 in 17
General population risk of colorectal cancer	1 in 35

In general, the following current guidelines for screening are used, with the frequency varying according to the level of risk.

History	Screening starts	Frequency
FAP	12–13 years	Yearly
HNPCC	Start 25 years (or 5 years before earliest age of diagnosis in the family)	≤ 2 yearly
Two 1st degree relatives affected One 1st degree relative < 45 years One 1st degree relative + two others on same side	Start at 5 years younger than mean age of cases	5 yearly (3 yearly if polyps seen)

Screening for colon cancer using fecal occult blood testing kits is now offered in some countries to those at population risk, but this is not a substitute for colonoscopic screening in those at higher than population risk.

10.2.4 Genetic counseling for familial cancer risk

When a family is referred because of a perceived risk of familial cancer, it is extremely important to document the family history accurately and confirm the diagnoses of cancer whenever possible.

Consent to view medical records of living family members is required from the individual concerned, but it may not be required to search the records of individuals who have died. However, in some countries it is necessary to obtain the permission of the next of kin to access the deceased's records. In the initial stage of the contact, forms may be given to the referred person to help them obtain the relevant information and to document the written consent from their relatives.

Cancer registries exist in many countries (for example the US, UK, Ireland, Australia, the Netherlands, Canada, and Iceland) and these are very useful places to obtain confirmation of cancer diagnoses, but in some cases medical records or death certificates are used. After confirmation of as many cases as possible, the risk to the referred person can be discussed, and recommendations for screening made.

10.2.5 Pre-symptomatic and predictive genetic testing in familial cancer

In both familial breast and bowel cancer, there may be a number of potential genes involved, and the mutation may differ from family to family. It is therefore necessary to identify the faulty gene in each family before genetic testing can be offered to unaffected family members. Samples from an affected person are required for analysis, and only when the gene mutation is found can pre-symptomatic or predictive testing be offered to others in the family. Our knowledge of the genetic causes of cancer has not yet progressed to the point where the mutation can be found in every family, and so some individuals who would like to know their status are unable to be tested.

If a person does request testing, and the mutation is known in the family, then the counselor works with the client to help him or her to prepare for the result. The preparatory counseling usually occupies two or three sessions at least.

Following the result, clients are generally followed up for some time, whatever the outcome. Those who are shown to have inherited the mutation will of course be advised to continue with their screening program. In some cases, clients who know they carry the gene mutation may opt for prophylactic surgery, such as mastectomy or oopherectomy. This is especially true of women who have experienced the loss of close relatives with breast and/or ovarian cancer, and who may be very concerned about leaving their own families without a mother.

There is evidence that women are more likely to communicate about health matters within a family, and to take the responsibility for informing others of risk. When a mother dies, her children may lose the person who would have been their main informant on these matters, although grandmothers and aunts often take over this role. For health professionals, it is helpful to be aware of the potential gap in health-related information that may exist in these families.

Collins Family

Carol Collins was diagnosed with colorectal cancer, and had a total colectomy when she was 29 years old. The histology report indicated multiple polyps in the section of bowel examined. The presence of hundreds of polyps in her bowel is diagnostic of FAP. Carol's mother Peggy died at 44 years of age with colon cancer, and it is likely she also had FAP, although the histology records are not available and the cancer registry records only the diagnosis of colon cancer. Carol says her mother was 'too far gone' for treatment when she was diagnosed.

As it is likely that the diagnosis in this family is FAP, those at risk in the family should be offered colonoscopic screening. Adam, Carol's oldest son is now 11 years of age. There are two other children in the family, Joe who is 8 years old and Amy who is 4.

Carol's brother Robert (27) has been suffering some rectal bleeding. Another sister, Miriam is only 18 years and has never been screened.

A blood sample is taken from Carol for genetic testing. Initially, a mutation is not found, so testing cannot be offered to Miriam or Robert. However, since they are at risk, they are urged to consider colonoscopic screening. Robert is reluctant, but finally agrees after pressure from his girlfriend. He does not turn up for the screening appointment.

Miriam has a colonoscopy and no polyps are found, which indicates she is unlikely to have inherited the gene mutation as some polyps would have been expected to have grown by the age of 18. She is, however, asked to return for screening again in 2 years.

Robert is encouraged by her result and goes for screening. He has multiple polyps and a small malignancy in the colon. An emergency colectomy is performed, but further therapy is not needed.

Several months later, the gene mutation is found in Carol's sample, and her brother and sister are tested. Miriam's test confirms she did not inherit the mutation and she requires no further screening. Miriam is both relieved and guilty about having 'escaped' the family condition. Robert has inherited the mutation, and his two children are at 50% risk themselves. This creates another challenge within the family, as Robert has lost touch with their mother and is unable to inform her that their children are at risk.

10.2.6 *Psychological implications of risk status*

One of the roles of the health professional is to encourage clients who are at high risk to use all the means available to increase their chances of survival, whether this is by self-examination, self-reporting or undergoing clinical investigation. Providing education on effective techniques for breast self-examination, or information on the potential signs and symptoms of bowel cancer is well within the remit of the primary care team, or nurses working in secondary care in a surgical team, for example.

There are many people at increased risk of cancer who seek clinical screening and who find reassurance in the knowledge that they are doing all they can to detect early cancer. However, in some cases the fear of discovering a tumor is so great that it impedes the person's ability to comply with screening. Lynch and Lynch [86] described this scenario in families at risk of bowel cancer, where the fear is overwhelming and therefore the client will not attend for colonoscopy. This is certainly evident in clinical practice. There are also many women at high risk of breast cancer who do not examine their own breasts regularly due to the fear of discovering a lump.

10.2.7 *The role of intrusion and avoidance*

The psychological concepts of intrusion and avoidance[86] are helpful in understanding responses to risk. Some women report examining their breasts regularly for a period of time after they are reminded of their risk, for example, after seeing the genetic counselor, or after another member of the family has a 'scare'. At those times, the cancer risk 'intrudes' into the thoughts frequently. However, intrusion is difficult to maintain, and the mind's response to constant intrusion is avoidance. Gradually, when the intrusion lessens, and the risk is less prominent, the motivation to self-examine is reduced.

The motivation to self-examine may be increased if the woman has encouragement from the primary care nurse, especially if the nurse is able to allocate time to meet with the woman regularly, perhaps once or twice a year, to check the breasts and discuss any concerns.

When a client continually fails to attend for screening, the reasons for such non-attendance may be complex. This is especially so if the client confirms the need for screening, makes appointments, but does not attend. As stated above, it may be fear of a tumor being discovered that prevents attendance, but there may also be other reasons.

Collins Family

Robert is at risk of FAP, and has rectal bleeding. He agrees to have a colonoscopy but does not turn up for the appointment. Robert has met the genetic counselor several times and she visits him at home a week later. He is reluctant to say why he did not attend. After a long conversation, Robert finally admits that he has spent time in prison, during which he was assaulted by an inmate. His fear of colonoscopy stems from this experience of anal rape.

10.3 Huntington disease – a model for pre-symptomatic testing

10.3.1 Description of Huntington disease

Huntington disease (HD) is a condition that affects the physical, mental, emotional and social health of the affected person. It has been known, since George Huntington first described the condition in the literature in 1872, that the disease is dominantly inherited, but until the mutation was identified in 1993 the concept of '**anticipation**' was puzzling. 'Anticipation' refers to the phenomenon in which succeeding generations of the family develop the disease at a younger age than the preceding generation. In families affected by HD, anticipation sometimes occurs, but sometimes not.

The mutation in the *huntingtin* gene is an expansion, that is, abnormal genes are longer than the normal gene. In the genetic material, certain base-pair sequences are often repeated within a gene. Within the *huntingtin* gene, unaffected individuals have up to 35 repeated copies of the sequence 'CAG'. However, affected patients have more than 35 copies of the CAG triplet in one copy of the gene. They thus have one normal and one expanded copy of the gene.

The CAG **trinucleotide** codes for glutamine, and the expanded gene increases the length of a glutamine chain in the cell cytoplasm, causing it to form clumps and invade the nucleus of the cell. This results in premature death of brain cells.

Once the number of CAG repeats in the gene has expanded, it is less stable and the number of repeats can increase when the gene is copied during meiosis. The expansion is more likely to increase during spermatogenesis than oogenesis. Hence if a man has HD, his children may inherit a larger copy of the gene than he has, and develop the condition at an earlier age than he did.

The age of onset is related to the size of the expanded fragment in the gene, and varies from childhood (rare) to the eighth or even ninth decade. However, the majority of people are diagnosed in their 40s.

The signs and symptoms of HD vary with each individual, but fall into three main groups.

- *Physical disability*. The first physical signs may be clumsiness, stumbling, and unsteadiness. Clients often see a deterioration in their handwriting, may trip when walking, and may spill drinks or food more frequently than usual. Eventually, chorea may be evident, and walking becomes very difficult. The speech becomes slurred.
- *Mental disability*. Initially, the client is often aware that their memory is becoming worse, especially their short-term memory. Ability to do mental arithmetic can also deteriorate and this can be evident when shopping. The 'executive functions' suffer, and clients will often find it hard to problem-solve or respond to changes in plans or situations. Some clients eventually suffer serious dementia.
- *Psychiatric problems*. Depression may be the first sign of HD, and can be effectively treated with anti-depressants. Paranoia and obsessive behavior may also be present; these are naturally difficult for the family to deal with, but can also be treated by the psychiatric team. Suicide is a significant risk.

10.3.2 *Pre-symptomatic testing*

For some people at risk, the uncertainty of their situation is difficult to bear, and they choose to have a pre-symptomatic test. This type of test is performed on a sample from a healthy individual to determine whether or not the person has inherited the gene mutation that will eventually cause the signs and symptoms of HD.

Prior to the test being available, studies showed that the majority of those at risk would request a test, but these results are not borne out by the actual uptake of predictive testing. However, less than one-quarter of those at risk actually request testing. This is understandable given that there are no preventative measures that could delay the onset of the disease, no cure and no effective treatment. Most people prefer to retain some hope that they have not inherited the condition.

A protocol for pre-symptomatic testing has been in use in the UK and many genetic centers worldwide since testing commenced[87]. This protocol is aimed at ensuring that clients who are tested have adequate opportunity to explore the implications for themselves and their families, and to prepare for either result. The test is only performed with informed consent.

Some of those who come forward for discussion about testing do so at the instigation of their family or health carers. However, the aim of the preparatory discussions is to help the client decide whether certainty is preferable to uncertainty, even if they receive 'bad news'.

For those who do decide that certainty is preferable, several counseling sessions are offered to help the client prepare for the result. The client is encouraged to bring a support person to the sessions, and is helped to plan the period following the results. Interestingly, those who have lived with the risk of HD for a number of years often find it difficult to adapt psychologically to not being at risk, as this appears to require a greater adjustment than finding out they are going to be affected. Many also suffer from survivor guilt, particularly if their siblings are affected. Strong emotional support is often required after the test, whatever the outcome, and when the result is good this is more often lacking because friends and family cannot understand why the client is having difficulties.

Harding Family

Mary is 50 years old, and the daughter of Cyril Harding. Cyril was diagnosed with Huntington disease when he was 50 years of age. He had been with the same firm since leaving school, working as an electrician and though he was unable to continue his normal work, they found a less demanding job for him in the stores department. He managed to work for 5 years after diagnosis, then took early retirement. He died at 62 years of age of pneumonia after breaking his hip in a fall.

Mary started showing some signs of HD in her late 30s, although it wasn't diagnosed until she was 41 years old. At that time she had a CT brain scan that showed significant changes.

Mary gave up work on at 43 years of age. She said it was all becoming too high-powered at the garden center where she worked. Everyone had to learn to use a new barcode system and she just couldn't get the hang of it, and anyway her husband made enough to keep them comfortable, especially once the kids had left home.

Mary has never had a genetic test, never saw the need for it, she knew she was just like Dad. It didn't seem fair though, that she got it so much earlier than him.

Cathy is Mary's daughter, and the granddaughter of Cyril Harding. Cathy is now 26 years old, and has known about her risk of HD since her mother was diagnosed about 9 years ago. It was a great shock to learn about the family condition at that time, and Cathy has broken off several relationships rather than tell a boyfriend about her risk.

Now Cathy has met a man she really loves, and told him about the HD after he met her family. Naturally he could see her mother was ill, as she uses a wheelchair and he had trouble understanding what she was saying to him.

Cathy and Tom plan to get married, and would like a family. They come to see the genetic counselor to discuss HD, and the risks to their future children. Together they decide that if Cathy has the gene they will get married, but will not have any children.

Before testing Cathy, the counselor visits Mary to ask if she can have a sample of blood to confirm that HD is the correct diagnosis. Mary enjoys the attention, and gives her consent for her sample to be tested. The test shows that Mary has one copy of the gene with 19 CAG repeats, and one copy with 45 repeats.

After three counseling sessions, Cathy has blood taken. Two weeks later she and Tom meet the counselor for the result to be given in person. Sadly, Cathy has inherited HD from her mother. She and Tom are distraught, but feel they have the information they need to plan their lives together with more certainty.

Three months later Cathy and Tom marry. It is a happy occasion, although afterwards Cathy finds it very hard to watch the video of her mother.

One year later Cathy rings the counselor to say that she and Tom have decided to have a family after all and she is pregnant.

The protocol developed for use in HD testing is also used for pre-symptomatic or predictive testing in other genetic conditions, such as CADASIL, myotonic dystrophy, adult polycystic kidney disease, and HNPCC. It is a useful model to use whenever the results of a test would give the client information about their future health, changing what is for them a potential situation into a certainty.

KEY PRACTICE POINT

A pre-symptomatic test could be defined as any test that changes a potential health risk for the client into a certainty. This does not just apply to genetic tests, but could apply in many 'screening' situations, such as a renal ultrasound that detects cysts, or a full blood count that could detect sickle cell disease. Clients should be supported when undergoing such tests, and prepared for possible outcomes.

10.3.3 *Care of people affected by HD*

The needs of clients affected by HD are diverse and require the input of professionals from many disciplines. A study[88] of affected individuals in a regional area showed that there were significant problems associated with communication between families and professionals in health and social care. Whilst some services were deficient, in many cases they existed but were accessed only after a crisis had occurred. A model of care that was introduced involves inter-disciplinary working, but the identification of a named key professional is crucial to the success of such teamwork. The key worker takes responsibility for the communication of information from one professional to another, for the regular assessment of the client's needs and for the organization of services at an early stage to reduce the necessity for crisis management, with all its inherent stresses on both the family and the services.

Harding Family

Peter Harding has been affected with HD for at least 6 years, although even before he was diagnosed he was very moody and prone to bouts of depression. These contributed to the divorce from his wife, before the reason was known.

Peter's ex-wife Angie now offers him a lot of support, but she lives two miles from him, and has a job to support their two children. For two or three years Peter met virtually no-one from week to week. However, after he set fire accidentally to the kitchen curtains while having a fry-up late one night, social services became aware of his needs. He now attends a day center three days a week, where he does gardening and cooking and plays computer games. He also has therapy every week at the center to help him with his speech and swallowing difficulties.

10.4 Psychiatric conditions

10.4.1 *Genetic influence on psychiatric conditions*

The knowledge of genetic influences on psychiatric conditions has altered dramatically over the past 10 years. Because of the disabling effect of psychiatric illness on everyday living, the difficult social effects on the family, and the stigma that is still attached to such conditions, family members are often very concerned about the risk that such conditions 'may be passed on'.

Assessing the genetic influence on such conditions is difficult. These disorders are relatively common in the general population, with a lifetime risk of around 1% for either affective disorder or schizophrenia[89]. As they follow no clear Mendelian patterns of inheritance, they are obviously not due simply to an inherited gene mutation. In addition, it is possible that being raised by a parent with a psychiatric condition may influence the mental health of the offspring of that family, making it more likely that there are multiple cases within a family. Studies of twins raised together or separately have shown that the children of parents with affective disorder and schizophrenia are more likely to develop these conditions than the offspring of unaffected parents.

10.4.2 *Affective disorder (manic-depression)*

This is a term used to cover manic depression or depression alone. Studies indicate that the earlier the age at which a person is affected, the more likely it is that relatives will also be affected. However, the only basis we have upon which to advise a client enquiring about their own risk is the empirical data collected on families. These data enable a risk figure to be given, ranging from a risk of 5% if a second degree relative has manic depression, to a risk of about 50% if both parents of the client have been affected.

10.4.3 *Schizophrenia*

Using data from empirical studies, it is clear that there is an increased risk of schizophrenia developing in relatives of an affected person. The genetic link is demonstrated when we consider the incidence of schizophrenia in twins. When one twin is affected, 40% of monozygotic twin siblings are also affected, as compared with only 10% of dizygotic twin siblings. This indicates that even after allowing for a common environment, the concordance for risk between those who inherit identical genetic material is high.

Again, the risk is high (45%) if both parents of the client have schizophrenia. It is important when advising families of their risk to try to confirm the diagnosis in the affected person. Some inherited neurological conditions such as Huntington disease or DRPLA may present with a severe psychiatric illness, but of course the risk to the client may be very different.

10.4.4 *Pre-senile dementia (early Alzheimer's disease)*

Pre-senile dementia is a condition (like breast or bowel cancer) that may occur sporadically, or may be caused by a gene mutation. Generally, late onset Alzheimer's disease will be due to old age, rather than an inherited mutation, but if there is a history of dementia occurring in several younger members of a family, this may be connected with a mutation in one of the presenilin genes. Where a gene mutation exists, children of an affected parent will be at 50% risk of inheriting the mutation and developing early dementia.

10.5 Genetic hemochromatosis

It is useful to look in detail at a recessive genetic condition that is detectable and where effective treatment is possible. The opportunity to treat a condition changes the rationale for testing pre-symptomatically. To help you think about some of the issues, we are going to work through the case of the Jones family.

CASE EXAMPLE   **JONES FAMILY**

Anne Jones rings up the genetics department in a great deal of distress. Her husband Mike is terminally ill with liver cancer. She is very angry because he had been complaining for some years of always being tired, pains in the joints in his fingers and generally feeling unwell. She said their life together had been very difficult over that time and one of her biggest regrets was that he had become impotent and this made her

---

feel that their marriage was in danger of being over even though she still loved him. She and Mike had always felt that he was ill but no diagnosis had been made until he became jaundiced and was shown to have liver cancer. He was then told he had hemochromatosis, a genetic disorder of iron metabolism that meant he carried on absorbing iron from his food even when he had sufficient iron stored in his body. This iron overload had probably caused his symptoms and had also led to the development of his liver cancer. The reason Anne was so angry, however, was that she had now been told that if Mike had been diagnosed with hemochromatosis before his liver damage had started, his cancer could have been prevented by the simple treatment of having blood taken regularly. She had been onto the internet and read that hemochromatosis was a common genetic disease, that it was recessive, and that one in ten people from Northern Europe carried the gene. She had worked out that if she also carried the gene, then her children were at a one in two chance of having the condition. She had to know if she carried the gene because she did not want her children to die of this terrible condition. She was also worried about Mike's sister and brother and had told them to go to their GP and be tested.

Think about how you would feel in this situation. What things would you want to know about before you had a test? If you were Mike's brother would you be anxious to be tested?

Some time later James, a cousin of Mike's, is seen in the genetic center. As a result of extended family testing he has been shown to have two copies of the gene mutation that gives a risk of hemochromatosis and has been referred to discuss the risk to his children. He is fit and well, his GP has checked his ferritin and transferrin saturation and he shows no evidence of iron overload. He is also angry, and walks into the counseling session saying that he wished he never heard of the condition; he was absolutely fine, but because he had had the test for hemochromatosis he was having trouble getting life insurance. No one could tell him if he was going to run into problems with this disease, or how many times he should see a doctor, or how often he should have blood tests done. In fact, the information he had been given was no use at all and he should never have had the test done.

Put yourself in James' position. What do you think about being tested for this condition now?

Genetic hemochromatosis is an autosomal recessive inherited disorder of iron metabolism. It is a treatable adult onset disorder and screening is possible either using measures of serum iron, transferrin saturation (the most sensitive measure), or using a genetic test.

The gene (*HFE*) was identified in 1996[90] and two common mutations account for 90% of cases in the European population. Most affected people have two copies of a mutation called C282Y, and a small proportion have the C282Y mutation together with a mutation called H63D. The genetic predisposition leads to accumulation of iron stored in the body over time.

Complications including cirrhosis, primary liver cancer, cardiomyopathy, arthritis and diabetes develop when iron overload is sufficient to cause organ damage[91]. Treatment for the condition involves removing multiple units of blood until the body iron stores return to normal. A maintenance program of venesection is then needed to prevent reaccumulation of iron. This treatment prolongs survival in symptomatic people and appears to restore normal life expectancy if started early enough in the course of the disease[92]. For this reason arguments have been made proposing population screening as a way of diagnosing this disease early and preventing its complications.

If we consider the *Case example* on the previous page, someone in Anne's position might be very positive about universal screening for hemochromatosis. If her husband had been diagnosed early enough then his cancer would have been prevented and he would not be dying. However, population screening requires a stringent analysis of potential costs and benefits because it involves taking a population who have no medical complaints and identifying some who may become ill. The main problem with screening for hemochromatosis is that the natural history of the condition is not known. It is clear that individuals identified both by screening for abnormal iron metabolism (transferrin saturation) or by using a DNA-based test do not inevitably develop complications from having the predisposition. The true risk of developing serious complications is not known. In addition, it is not clear what strategy should be used for screening, biochemical or genetic, or when and how screening programs should be carried out. There is also legitimate concern about possible 'genetic discrimination', that is, effects on insurance and employment, for example, if an individual is identified as having the predisposition for developing this condition. For this reason, population screening is not recommended at the present time. However, genetic hemochromatosis could prove to be an important problem in which to consider the possible positive and negative effects of using genetic testing to identify disease predisposition for the purpose of treatment or prevention.

10.6 The perspective of the family carer

While family members and friends may take a role in caring for any person with a genetic condition, the impact of caring may be most pronounced when the family member is affected by an adult-onset condition. In this case, the person with the condition may have to discontinue working and may also have dependent children. This means that the responsibility for supporting the family financially and raising the children, as well as the tasks involved in caring for the affected person, may fall to the partner or other family members.

There is much literature on what is described as the 'burden' of caring. While some people undoubtedly find care-giving difficult and stressful, other carers find it offensive when it is assumed that they find the role burdensome. They are keen to point out that being a carer for a loved relative offers them positive benefits, including a sense of fulfilment and feelings associated with being needed.

In recent studies focusing on the needs of family carers, those who had a spouse or partner with a long-term condition described the loneliness they felt in having to make all the decisions, even the most basic ones. Neurodegenerative diseases, such as Huntington disease, may affect not only the behavior of the affected person, but also their ability to empathize with others. One of the hardest issues cited by carers in one study[93] was the lack of concern and appreciation for all they were doing. In some cases, carers said that the only way they could cope with the changes was to cease seeing the person as a partner and view them more as an additional child for whom they were responsible. Worry about the financial and practical aspects of care caused them concern. They also reported feeling very unsupported by professionals who did not understand the needs of the affected person. The multiplicity of health and social care services needed also required huge energy to organize. In thinking about the needs of people with a genetic condition, it is important to realize that the carer may have personal needs for support that may even conflict at times with the needs of the affected person. Specific support for carers, addressing their own needs, is essential to reduce avoidable damage to the carer's physical and mental health.

10.7 The multi-professional team and long-term care

We have been discussing a number of conditions in this chapter that require long-term supportive care for the affected person. Because a change in a single gene can have an effect on the cells in many parts of the body, genetic conditions often involve multiple body systems. Consideration needs to be given at an early stage with regard to the types of professionals who may be able to contribute positively to the care of the individual. For example, a person with von Hippel–Lindau disease may benefit from the expertise of people working in the fields of neurology, ophthalmology, urology, social work and genetics, while a person with Marfan syndrome will require some input from professionals in cardiology, cardiac surgery, orthopedics, ophthalmology and genetics. These services may be provided via a comprehensive care center or via multiple organizations. Whichever model is used, it is essential to appoint a key worker who acts as a co-ordinator for the multiplicity of services involved. This is often a specialist nurse, but it is more important that the person appointed is able to work closely with the family and to communicate well with all other partners in the multi-professional team.

10.8 Informed consent and mental capacity

The need to obtain informed consent for any procedure or genetic test has been covered in *Chapter 1*. However, when the client or patient is an adult with a learning disability or dementia, specific challenges may arise in ensuring that informed consent is given. As the applications of genetics and genomics increase across the health services, it will be more common to offer a test with a genetic basis to all people in the general population. For example, it may be relevant to offer patients a **pharmacogenomic** test to ascertain the best type or dosage of medication, and it would be inequitable to withhold such testing from people affected by dementia or learning disability. It should be assumed that the person with the learning disability is capable of giving consent, unless it is shown to be otherwise. In each country, practitioners should make themselves familiar with the legal requirements for practice in this area; for example, the Mental Capacity Act[94] in the UK states that another adult cannot give consent on behalf of the client or patient.

The ability to give consent may vary according to each situation, as it relates to the person, (i) having the appropriate information to make the decision, (ii) understanding the information, and (iii) being able to communicate their decision to either give or withhold consent. In addition, as obtaining consent is a process, rather than a single act, you may need to revisit the issue at each meeting to ensure that the person is still consenting. It may also be useful to include a person trusted by the client in any discussions (with the client's permission) as someone who knows the person well may be more likely to be able to assess whether they have understood the information.

10.9 Conclusion

In this chapter, we have described the influence of genes on three very different types of adult-onset disease. Genetic hemochromatosis is treatable if detected in the early stages, whilst screening and early treatment can influence the outcome for those at high risk of familial cancer. At present there is no cure for HD and other neurodegenerative disorders.

Psychological care of adult patients is as important as genetic information, as guilt, blame, anxiety and hopelessness may accompany the feeling of risk in any of these situations. As expressed earlier, it is not necessarily the risk but the perceived burden of the disease that is important to the family. Adults with first-hand experience of a disease will perceive it differently from those who have only been told about the condition by others. The use of counseling skills in any genetic situation helps the practitioner to understand the client's perspective and therefore to offer appropriate support.

Test yourself

Q1. A woman attending her GP surgery is aware of the risk of breast and ovarian cancer. She accepts mammographic screening for herself but does not wish to tell her sisters of the risk. How could the professionals involved in her care approach this situation? Do you believe that they have a duty of care to her siblings? What is the legal situation with respect to sharing information with a patient's relatives in your own country?

Q2. Is it worthwhile undertaking genetic tests for a man whose father had genetic hemochromatosis? Explain your response.

Q3. Prenatal testing for a mutation in the MLH2 gene (a gene fault that predisposes to colon cancer) is possible in some families with a history of HNPCC (hereditary non-polyposis colon cancer). In your opinion, is termination of pregnancy because of an increased risk of bowel and endometrial cancer in adulthood appropriate? What factors might influence a couple to request prenatal testing for an adult-onset familial cancer such as HNPCC?

Further resources

www.hda.org.uk/ – Huntington's Disease Association.

www.hdsa.org/ – Huntington's Disease Society of America.

www.huntington-assoc.com/ – International Huntington Association.

www.nature.com/scitable/topicpage/Tumor-Suppressor-TS-Genes-and-the-Two-887 – Chial H (2008) Tumor suppressor (TS) genes and the two-hit hypothesis. *Nature Education*, **1**. *A good description of the Knudson two-hit hypothesis.*

www.nice.org.uk/Guidance/CG41 – National Institute for Health and Clinical Excellence (NICE). *Information for patients on familial breast cancer.*

www.nice.org.uk/nicemedia/pdf/CG041PublicInfoCorrected.pdf – National Institute for Health and Clinical Excellence (NICE). *Guidelines on risk assessment and recommended screening for individuals with family history of breast or breast/ovarian cancer.*

www.opsi.gov.uk/ACTS/acts2005/ukpga_20050009_en_1 – Mental Capacity Act (2005).

Bennett RL (1999) *The Practical Guide to the Genetic Family History.* New York: Wiley-Liss. *Detailed information, especially on cancer syndromes.*

Lalloo F, Kerr B, Friedman J, Evans G (2005) *Risk assessment and management in cancer genetics.* Oxford: Oxford University Press.

Older adulthood

11.1 Introduction

In the last few years it has become apparent that the science of genomics has much to contribute to our understanding of aging and may contribute to enhanced healthcare for individuals in the later stages of life. In this chapter, we will discuss topics such as the effect of genes in aging, genetic influences on dementia and cancer, the use of pharmacogenomics in prescribing drugs for treatment of common diseases, and the attitudes of the elderly towards genomics-based testing.

Aging has been defined by Yunis et al.[95] as 'the genetically programmed decline in the functional effectiveness of an organism'. The term 'senescence' is used to describe the increase in mortality due to aging[96]. Longevity of any organism is limited by the changes in cells, tissues or systems that occur in the process of aging. The rate of change is affected by genetic, environmental and cultural factors. There has been considerable work undertaken on the contribution of genomic factors to aging. For example, are there different genetic variations that contribute to premature aging in some individuals or that enable the 'super-elderly' to continue active lives past the age of 100 years? Some research conducted on the development of neurodegenerative disease and premature aging in the rare inherited diseases has informed this work, but there is now a huge body of work focusing solely on the genomics of aging.

11.2 Genomics and aging

It is not possible to include in this book a comprehensive account of the work on genomic influences on aging and senescence. However, we are summarizing a few relevant examples here to provide the health professional with an idea of the range of current research.

Immunosenescence is a term used to describe the way in which the function of the immune system deteriorates over time[97]. This deterioration contributes to both morbidity and mortality in older adults because it can induce a chronic state of inflammation. Genetic variants that help to balance the pro- and anti-inflammatory processes in the body appear to act in a protective way against this condition, known as inflammaging[97].

In work on neurodegeneration in the aged population, genes that control the function of a proteosome called 26S have been found to have an impact on the rate of aging[98]. The gradual loss of this proteosome in the cells over the person's lifetime reduces the protection against unfolded or misfolded proteins in the neural cells. This may result in accumulation of polyglutamine that suppresses neurological function, similar to the process that occurs in genetic conditions such as Huntington disease.

Studies[99] on cardiovascular disease in older adults have also indicated that those individuals who inherit a particular variant of a gene (cholesteryl ester transfer protein gene, or *CETP*) that influences high-density lipoprotein cholesterol levels are more likely to live longer. This is thought to be because the variant (Int 14A) is associated with higher levels of this type of cholesterol, which seems to confer protection against a number of age-related diseases.

11.2.1 *Genomics, aging and cancer*

As apoptosis occurs throughout the lifespan, new cells develop from the pool of stem cells in a particular organ. As was described in *Chapter 10*, mutations in those cells can influence the development of cancer. With age, the pool of potential stem cells is reduced and the quality of the stem cells may therefore be less than ideal. This can explain the increasing chance of developing cancer with increasing age. Some authors suggest that exposure to toxins or mutagens in fetal life or early in infancy can alter the quality of the available stem cells, making some individuals more prone to develop cancer later in their lifetimes[100].

Another influence on aging has been found to be due to the action of a set of proteins called the RecQ helicases[101]. These are highly conserved across species and have a role in protecting the integrity of the DNA during replication, recombination and repair. For example, some helicases have been shown to guard against errors in recombination during mitosis. Mutations in the helicase genes can therefore indirectly predispose to the development of cancer, because they fail to prevent somatic mutations in genes that may themselves work to prevent the formation of cancer.

11.3 Genetic testing and common diseases

When considering rare inherited conditions, there is a strong link between a genetic mutation and the subsequent development of a disease. However, it is increasingly clear that individuals inherit one or more polymorphisms that give them a higher or lower chance of developing more common diseases, such as coronary heart disease, cancer or Parkinson disease. There has been much interest in genetic testing to predict risk of common diseases. Enthusiasm about the potential of such testing was raised, particularly during the period in which the Human Genome Project was being conducted. This major multi-national collaborative study culminated in the sequencing of the entire human genome[24]. However, it appears that in practice, testing for susceptibility for common diseases is less likely to be helpful in clinical healthcare than was expected. As was shown in the preceding section, while there have been genetic factors identified in many diseases, the actual development of the condition also depends upon environmental factors that may or may not be controllable. For example, Parkinson disease is a neurological condition occurring in about 5% of people who live beyond the age of 85 years[100]. Studies of the etiology of Parkinson disease have yet to identify a single gene that is responsible for the condition, yet there do appear to be genetic components implicated in the disease and it is regarded as a multi-factorial condition that is caused by a combination of both genetic and environmental factors (including exposure to toxins). In reality, testing for a combination of genetic variants that would indicate a person has a predisposition to one or more diseases may be no more helpful (and possibly less helpful) than monitoring their weight, diet, physical activity and use of substances. While for some people the knowledge that they have an increased genetic predisposition to a disease may influence them to try to reduce other risk factors, others may take the approach that they are bound to get the condition anyway, so why should they worry about lifestyle measures. In this sort of situation, the positive and negative benefits of knowing the information need to be carefully weighed. This should include addressing issues such as whether the test result gives any useful information about possible treatment, what the costs and benefits of the treatment are, and whether behavior change could have an impact. In addition, because this is a genetic test, the individual needs to consider whether the test result could have implications for the rest of the family.

11.4 Pharmacogenomics

Pharmacogenomics targets drug therapy to those patients for whom a particular medication will have the greatest effect. Traditionally, medicines were developed to treat signs and symptoms of a condition. Where different medications were available, the patient tried these until a satisfactory option was found, and the correct therapeutic dosage was ascertained through trial and error. This of course means that a proportion of patients will be treated with drugs that have no beneficial effect for them, or that produce unwanted side-effects or complications. The science of pharmacogenomics is based on the principle that genes control the production of enzymes that metabolize drugs. In *Chapter 4*, it was explained that all humans have genetic variation. If a variation in the usual sequence of base pairs occurs in over 1% of the population, this is called a polymorphism, and is considered to be a normal variant. Variation in certain genes which have an influence on the metabolism of drugs affects the individual's response to that drug.

In appropriate situations, testing a patient for genetic variation prior to prescribing a drug will enable the right drug to be administered in the right dose. As older adults are more likely to suffer from diseases that are treated with medication, they may benefit most from pharmacogenomics. A simple genetic test to look at the polymorphic variation present in the patient will provide the information needed to target the drug. We include here some relevant examples where testing for a gene variant prior to commencing therapy would identify those who are likely to respond well and those patients who will receive little or no benefit from the medication:

■ variants in specific apolipoproteins that are known to affect lipoprotein metabolism (APOA1/C3/A4/A5) have been shown to play a part in determining the way that patients respond to drug therapy to reduce triglyceride levels in the blood[102]

■ tamoxifen is frequently used therapeutically for women with breast cancer; polymorphisms of the *CYP2D6* gene have an impact on the clinical efficacy of the drug[103]

■ CYP2D6 and CYP2C19 are enzymes from the cytochrome group that influence the metabolism of anti-depressant medications[104]

■ a polymorphic variant of the *5-HTT* gene has been shown to have an influence on the likelihood of older adults becoming depressed and the efficacy of treatment using serotonin re-uptake inhibitors (SSRIs)[105].

While pharmacogenomic testing can already be useful in some specific clinical situations, it may be some time before it is used routinely in practice.

11.5 Attitudes of older adults to genetic testing

Whereas genetic testing may be possible to guide prescription of medication in the elderly, any innovation can only be introduced if it is acceptable to the population to whom it is offered. In order to assess the attitudes of older adults to the use of genomics in healthcare, focus groups were undertaken in the UK[106] and US[107]. Older adults (over 65 years of age) were invited to discuss their attitudes to genetic testing; they were keen to utilize any scientific advances available to them, as long as they felt that those responsible for their healthcare supported the use of such options. They were aware of the possible unethical practices carried out in the name of eugenics, but felt on the whole that they would trust their own healthcare professionals. When asked what they would require to give their consent to a genomics test, some wanted all possible information, while others felt they would wish to have information about the potential benefits of the test, for their own families or others. One interesting aspect of the approach of the older adults was that they were concerned about having to give the information resulting from a genomic test to their family members. They felt it would be preferable for others to relay any information that might have an impact on the family. This may indicate a sensitivity to be being blamed or simply not wishing to seen as the cause of anxiety to their relatives.

11.6 Psychosocial issues relevant to older adults

As has been described in many ways in this book, genetic conditions can have an impact well beyond the people affected. The effect of a genetic diagnosis in the family may well have a significant impact on the older members of the family. For example, a new diagnosis or the death of a young family member may trigger memories of similar losses in previous generations. These losses may have been dealt with in a very different way in the past, when pregnancy loss or the death of a newborn may not have been discussed openly, and unresolved grief can become apparent at the time of a new loss.

Older adults also express guilt at passing down a genetic mutation to the next generation, even when, as is often the case, they were unaware of this possibility. In the past, before genetic testing was possible, couples whose children were at risk of a genetic condition were frequently advised by health professionals not to have a family, and they may have been thought irresponsible for going ahead with a pregnancy. Because of stigmatization in the community, they may have felt they could not confide in others about their feelings. The psychological impact of long-term guilt and grief is sometimes very evident in the responses of the older generation of the family to the actions or decisions of younger relatives.

In practice, it is important to acknowledge the impact of many family situations on those of the older generation, whose current losses might be compounded by many other previous experiences.

Spencer Family

Luke Spencer has been diagnosed with fragile X syndrome. His mother Tracy has had carrier testing and is a carrier of this X-linked condition. There are female relatives on her mother's side of the family who may be at risk and the genetic counselor asks if she could bring Luke's grandmother (Sonia) to the next appointment so she can discuss carrier testing with her. If Sonia is not a carrier, there will be no need to offer testing for fragile X to her side of the family.

When Tracy broaches the subject with her mother, Sonia refuses to come to the appointment and will not talk about the issue. Tracy cannot understand her response, as she is very close to her daughter and adores her grandson. It is Tracy's father who tells her that Sonia's two brothers were put into an institution when she was young and she had been warned by her GP not to risk having a family. She feels guilty and is afraid that the genetic counselor will blame her for Luke's condition. If she is found to be a carrier, she fears Tracy will not forgive her and she will blame herself even more.

Tracy explains the situation to the counselor and together they decide that Tracy will speak to her cousins and offer them the chance to see the genetic counselor to discuss their possible risk. The counselor also offers to see Sonia if she wishes, but she does not accept the offer.

11.7 Conclusion

The use of genomics is increasingly relevant to healthcare of older adults. Practitioners should also be aware of the psychological impact of a genetic diagnosis in the family on the older generation and the influence of their previous experiences on their approaches to genetic testing.

Test yourself

Q1. Describe at least two discoveries that have informed our understanding of the influence of genes on the aging process.

Q2. Which group of genes are known to be involved in the metabolism of drugs used in the treatment of depression? Name two specific genes that are of significance.

Q3. In what way could a test for variation in an apolipoprotein gene influence treatment of an elderly person with high triglyceride levels contributing to cardiovascular disease?

Further resources

www.ama-assn.org/ama/pub/category/2306.html – American Medical Association information on pharmacogeneomics. *Includes scenarios and practical applications.*

www.ncbi.nlm.nih.gov/About/primer/pharm.html – NIH factsheet on pharmaco-genomics.

www.pharmgkb.org/ – Pharma Gkb information on pharmacogenomics. *Explanations of the underlying science of pharmacogenomics.*

12 Development of genetic healthcare competence in the health professions

12.1 Introduction

In this chapter we will provide some background to the development of genetic service and the health profession now known as genetic counseling. However, as genetic healthcare is provided by a wide range of practitioners, we will also address the core competences in genetics that are required by health professionals from primary and secondary care to provide safe care for patients.

Genetic services have developed as a specialist service in healthcare over the past 60 years. Clinical genetic services were established in both Europe and North America in the post-war period, but substantial growth occurred in the 1980s, as recombinant DNA technology opened the door to a number of new tests and services for families. The specific remit of genetic services is to provide information and support for individuals and families at risk of, or affected by, a genetic condition. In many countries (including the USA, Canada, the UK, The Netherlands, Belgium, Australia, and New Zealand), the service is provided by medical geneticists and non-medical genetic counselors or nurses working together in teams, and this model is being adapted increasingly in Europe and Asia.

12.2 A matter of peas – historic development in genetics

It is difficult to identify with any accuracy the birth of the profession of genetic counseling, but most people would acknowledge Gregor Mendel as the father of genetics. He spent years patiently breeding peas, counting the offspring, using the hybrids to produce more plants, and counting the resultant plants (see *Section 4.5*). His meticulous work led him to discover and describe accurately the mode of recessive inheritance. However, while Mendel laid the basis for genetic theory, it was Francis Galton who began to test the theories in relation to humans. Mendel and Galton were born the same year (1822). Mendel's scientific pursuits were somewhat restricted by his theological vocation, and perhaps by the lack of acknowledgement he received in his lifetime, whereas Galton became one of the Victorian polymaths. Galton was the cousin of Charles Darwin, and the publication in 1859 of *The Origin of Species*[108] had influenced his thoughts on matters of heredity and his religious beliefs. In the retrospective light of current scientific method, Galton's studies were primitive and naïve, however, perhaps the greatest value of Galton's work lies in his interest in the new territory of human genetics. His varied studies included work on the hereditary nature of ability[109,110] and the numerical assessment of risk[111]. Galton's interest in inherited traits continued to influence his scientific ventures, and eventually he realized that the traits were somehow inherited from both parents, and that they were transferred in the fertilized ovum. He experimented using sweet peas independently of Mendel, and performed twin studies.

The outcome of Galton's research and thinking on these matters was the development of the theory of eugenics. He proposed that as characteristics necessary for the improvement of the species are largely inherited, it made sense to encourage breeding of the 'fitter' members of a society, and to discourage those 'less fit' from having children. In this way any society could be enhanced, for whilst the struggle for survival applies equally to all species, the knowledge of inheritance confers upon man the opportunity to influence his own evolution. Galton regarded eugenics as a science in its own right, a theory which was morally superior to natural selection. He felt natural selection relied upon over-production and subsequent destruction of excessive stock. By enhancing conditions for reproduction of healthy stock, Galton felt that not only society, but the individuals within that society, would benefit[112]. This was a theory based on the belief that all those born into society ought to be able to make a positive contribution, thus resulting in a better society in the long term. However, it relied upon the subjective judgements of certain individuals (self-selected) about the worth of other individuals, and for that reason many people find it unacceptable.

12.3 The eugenics movement

The Eugenics Society was born of Galton's ideas. Although Galton emphasized the need for such judgement of human fitness to be based on statistical evidence, this type of evidence is unobtainable by ethical means. As Blacker[112], a prominent member of the Eugenics Society, later said, as both genetics and environment have an influence on the eventual ability of a person to contribute positively to society, the judgement can only be made where environmental influence is absolutely equal, therefore making such a judgement is impossible. Blacker also made the distinction that the Eugenics Society was occupied with the *study* rather than the *practice* of eugenics.

The eugenics movement certainly had its critics, one of the most vocal being GK Chesterton, who felt that the principles of eugenics increased the burden of the working class by inhibiting reproductive choice. At the time it was not only those with genetic conditions who were considered 'unfit' to breed. Many acquired medical conditions such as syphilis, tuberculosis and alcoholism were thought to be inherited; poverty, criminality and prostitution were also indicators of unfitness.

A Bill in the UK concerning voluntary sterilization for those in the Social Problem Group was drafted by the Brock Committee in 1934, but did not become legislation. One of the aims of the Eugenics Society[112] was to make affordable contraceptive methods available to those who wished to have them, but the Brock Committee legislation differed in that it was based on a judgement of fitness rather than personal choice.

The abhorrence of eugenic principles felt by some individuals was very probably exacerbated by the distortion and abuse of the original ideals by those with completely different motives from those of the founders of the Eugenics Society. The notoriety of eugenics reached a zenith during the period of the Third Reich in Germany in the 1930s. Hitler had stated his belief in the supremacy of the Aryan peoples in *Mein Kampf*, suggesting that the State had both a moral and practical responsibility to ensure that only those who were genetically desirable should procreate. This belief culminated in plans to sterilize sufferers and carriers of hereditary diseases. In 1933 a compulsory sterilization law was passed, which affected those people suffering from hereditary deafness, blindness and Huntington disease, among other congenital disabilities. Later in the same decade these disabilities became grounds for extermination under the same regime. However, compulsory sterilization for genetic disease has not been solely confined to Germany, it has also been practiced in the United States and in a number of Scandinavian countries[13].

12.4 Growth of medical genetics

The first episode of genetic counseling is said to have taken place in 1895[86], when a doctor discussed the risk of familial cancer with a seamstress who had a strong family history of the disease. The doctor reported that the seamstress looked sad, and when questioned she confessed that she felt her time on earth was limited, due to the frequent occurrence of cancer in her family. She proved to be right, dying young of the condition.

However, the importance of genetics to medicine only became generally appreciated with the discovery of the genetic basis of disease early in the twentieth century. One of the first publications on what would now be termed genetic counseling appeared in 1933, entitled *The Chances of Morbid Inheritance*. Blacker wrote the book to assist doctors in advising patients about the chances of having a child with an inherited condition. The emphasis was placed on informing couples on the *advisability* of having children. In view of the inability of medical science to detect problems prenatally, or to treat the majority of conditions, the options for couples at risk were limited. An extension of the Eugenic Society's work in this field occurred just prior to the Second World War, when it undertook to offer advice to people who were seeking information on their genetic risks, prior to marriage or having a family. However, the suspicion with which modern genetic counseling is viewed by some couples may have stemmed from these early connections with the eugenics movement.

One doctor who recognized the importance of genetics in disease causation was Archibald Garrod[113] who built upon Mendel's discoveries to determine the autosomal recessive inheritance of a number of conditions termed 'inborn errors of metabolism'. Garrod was able to predict correctly the 25% risk of inheriting the disease for children of two carrier parents. He also comprehended the relevance of consanguineous marriage to recessive inheritance of disease. In 1931, Lancelot Hogben, a Professor of Social Science, proposed the establishment of dedicated units for the study of human genetics, staffed by teams comprising geneticists, statisticians, doctors, psychologists and ethnologists. Hogben had grasped the complexity of the subject of clinical genetics and its probable influence on individual human existence. His call for qualified workers in a number of disciplines reflects the organization of many modern clinical genetic services.

12.5 Establishment of specialist clinical genetic services

The first clinical department of genetics in the UK was established at The Hospital for Sick Children, Great Ormond Street, London, and a geneticist was employed for clinical duties within the hospital from 1951. At the time it was believed that genetic services were needed to help parents to decide whether to have further children. Genetic specialists could also make other medical staff aware of the chance of an affected child being born, to facilitate early diagnosis and treatment[114].

Clinical genetic services are now a regular part of healthcare provision in many countries. Accurate human chromosomal studies have been possible since the late 1950s and these have enabled syndromes caused by chromosomal imbalance to be identified accurately. Further stimulus for expansion arrived with the advent of recombinant DNA technology in the 1970s. While clinical examination of patients is still important, gene mutation analysis is increasingly helpful in clarifying the genetic diagnosis, and making prenatal, pre-symptomatic and predictive testing available to families. Increasing awareness of the psychological impact of genetic conditions and risk upon families has led to the inclusion of psychological support as an integral part of genetic services.

12.6 Genetic services – the current situation

Clinical genetic services are currently involved with diagnosis of the condition, the prevention or amelioration of the disease, and information about risk and reproductive choice. Whilst the technology has enhanced the diagnostic skill, risk assessment, treatment and options, it appears that the underlying human rationale for the service has not been clouded by pure technology. However, it is clear that the forces influencing the development of clinical genetic services have derived first from an academic, and then from a medical model. The model of service has now been further modified due to the influence of genetic counselors, who see a primary part of their role as providing support to families.

While clinical genetics is established across Europe, North America, Australasia and Asia, the quality and type of service provision varies enormously. Most teams are led by medical geneticists, and in some areas medical personnel are the sole providers. For example, in some European countries, genetic services are provided almost exclusively by medical or laboratory staff with very little input from other professions such as nursing. However, in an increasing number of countries, other professionals such as genetic counselors, genetic nurses, or psychologists are employed within the team.

12.7 Establishment of a genetic counseling profession

The four main components of the role of genetic counselor are as follows.

- Communication with clients to obtain the family medical history necessary to provide the client with reliable information, convey the genetic information, and present the options available to the family in a non-judgemental manner.
- Client support, particularly at times of decision-making or particular stress, for example, after a new diagnosis has been made in the family, during an at-risk pregnancy, or when testing is being considered.
- Education of clients and other health professionals on issues related to clinical genetics.
- Skilled interpretation of current research findings for the benefit of clients.

It is apparent that the demand for genetic services will increase as technology offers more in the form of genetic testing, pharmacogenetics and possibly gene therapy. In addition to the rare genetic disorders, genetic services may also be required to make a contribution to the healthcare of those with common conditions in which there is a genetic component. This may not be direct care for patients with those conditions, but will almost certainly involve providing education and consultation for other healthcare professionals[115].

The genetic counselor needs to be educated sufficiently to interpret the complex scientific data for the benefit of patients, and to possess the counseling skills necessary to ensure clients can express their opinions, explore the options and make informed decisions. As genetic counseling is overwhelmingly a practical clinical exercise, training programs must include opportunities for observation of good practice and supervized clinical practice for the student.

Plasschaert et al.[116] defined competences as the set of behaviors that are expected by independent practitioners in particular professions. One method of ensuring that genetic counselors and nurses acquire the requisite standard of skills and knowledge to practice safely is to align training programs to a set of core competences. The EuroGentest project is a major research project aimed at harmonizing and standardizing genetic testing in Europe. It is acknowledged that many professionals will be involved in delivering genetic information to individuals and families. However, the EuroGentest project team recommends that genetic counseling is provided by a suitably prepared and qualified specialist in genetic counseling in specific situations, including pre-symptomatic and prenatal testing. An Expert Group working within the EuroGentest project has devised a set of core competences for genetic counselors and nurses working in Europe[117] (*Table 12.1*). This has been based

Table 12.1. Core competences for genetic nurses and genetic counselors in Europe

1. Establish relationship and clarify the counselee's concerns and expectations.
2. Make appropriate and accurate genetic risk assessment.
3. a. Convey clinical and genetic information to counselees, appropriate to their individual needs.
   b. Explain options available to the counselee, including the risks, benefits and limitations.
   c. Evaluate the understanding of the individual related to the topics being discussed.
   d. Acknowledge the implications of individual and family experiences, beliefs, values and culture for the genetic counseling process.
4. Make an assessment of counselees' needs and resources and provide support, ensuring referral to other agencies as appropriate.
5. Use of a range of counseling skills to facilitate counselees' adjustment and decision-making.
6. Document information including case notes and correspondence in an appropriate manner.
7. Find and utilize relevant medical and genetic information for use in genetic counseling.
8. Demonstrate ability to organize and prioritize a case load.
9. Plan, organize and deliver professional and public education
10. Establish effective working relationships to function within a multidisciplinary team and as part of the wider health and social care network.
11. Contribute to the development and organization of genetic services.
12. Practice in accordance with an appropriate code of ethical conduct.
13. Recognize and maintain professional boundaries and limitations of own practice.
14. Demonstrate reflective skills and personal awareness for the safety of individuals and families.
15. Present opportunities for clients to participate in research projects in a manner that facilitates informed choice.
16. Demonstrate continuing professional development as an individual practitioner and for the development of the profession.

upon other documents, such as the Standard and Scope of Practice for genetic nurses published by the International Society of Nurses in Genetics[118] and the core competences used by the Genetic Counsellor Registration Board (UK and Ireland) to assess candidates for registration as a genetic counselor[119]. The core competences and sets of suggested learning outcomes for each can be viewed at the EuroGentest website (see *Further resources*).

12.8 Core competences in genetics for health professionals not specializing in genetics

As has been demonstrated throughout this text, the use of genetics and genomics within a wide range of healthcare settings requires health professionals to develop sufficient knowledge and skills in genetics to enable them to practice safely and appropriately. The set of core competences[117] in *Table 12.2* is relevant to general nurses, such as those working in general practice, on general medical or surgical wards, in an acute care setting, or in general ambulatory medicine.

Table 12.2. Core competences in genetics for general nurses/midwives

1. Identify individuals who might benefit from genetic information and services.
2. Tailor genetic information and services to the individual's culture, knowledge and language.
3. Uphold the rights of all individuals to informed decision-making and voluntary action.
4. Demonstrate knowledge of the role of genetic and other factors in health and disease.
5. Demonstrate a knowledge and understanding of the utility and limitations of genetic testing and information.
6. Recognize the limitation of one's own genetic expertise.

The competences[117] included in *Table 12.3* are considered appropriate for those nurses or midwives who have a more specialist role, such as specialists in the hemoglobinopathies, fetal medicine, or oncology.

These competences are designed to be adaptable to a range of cultural, national, health and educational settings. Similar sets of competences exist for practitioners in other disciplines such as medicine or laboratory science.

Table 12.3. Core competences in genetics for specialist nurses, specialist midwives and specialist allied health professionals

1. Identify individuals who might benefit from genetic information and services.
2. Tailor genetic information and services to the individual's culture, knowledge and language.
3. Uphold the rights of all individuals to informed decision-making and voluntary action.
4. Demonstrate knowledge of the role of genetic and other factors in health and disease.
5. Demonstrate a knowledge and understanding of the utility and limitations of genetic testing and information.
6. Recognize the limitation of one's own genetic expertise.
7. Obtain and communicate credible current information about genetics for self, clients and colleagues.

12.9 Conclusion

The new profession of genetic counseling is becoming established to provide care, support and information for families at risk of a genetic condition. However, genetics is increasingly a core component of everyday healthcare, and professionals from many disciplines and specialties will need to be educated about genetics to work competently and confidently with clients. Skill in counseling, and an awareness of the potential ethical, psychological and social issues are necessary for competent practice and are all included in the core competences for health professionals.

Further resources

www.agnc.org.uk/Registration/registration.htm – Genetic Counsellor Registration Board (UK).

www.eshg.org/ – European Society of Human Genetics.

www.eurogentest.org/unit6/ – EuroGentest Unit 6 (Education) website. *Core competence documents.*

www.geneticseducation.nhs.uk/ – National Genetics Education and Development Centre (UK).

www.geneticseducation.nhs.uk/tellingstories/ – Telling Stories – Understanding Real Life Genetics. *Website featuring the stories of families affected by genetic conditions, linking each story to the core competences in genetics.*

www.isong.org/ – International Society of Nurses in Genetics.

www.nchpeg.org/ – National Coalition for Health Professional Education in Genetics (US).

www.nsgc.org – National Society of Genetic Counselor s (US).

www.nvgc.info/hoofdpagina%20e.htm – Dutch Association of Genetic Counselors NVGC (The Netherlands).

Glossary of terms

Affected individual: A person who has the signs and symptoms of the genetic condition.

Allele: A copy of the gene at a particular locus. One allele is inherited from each parent.

Amniocentesis: Withdrawal of amniotic fluid from the amniotic sac, usually for the purpose of testing the fetal chromosomes.

Anencephaly: Failure of the anterior neural tube to close properly during very early intrauterine life resulting in the absence of the cerebral hemispheres and skull bone together with a rudimentary brain stem.

Aneuploidy: An alteration in the number of chromosomes, involving only one or several chromosomes rather than the entire set of chromosomes.

Anticipation: The phenomena whereby successive generations of a family manifest a genetic condition more seriously or at a younger age.

Assisted reproduction: Any artificial technique used to enable a pregnancy to be achieved (e.g. *in vitro* fertilization).

Autism: A form of mental disability characterized by failure to interact with others.

Autosomal dominant inheritance pattern: The inheritance pattern whereby one copy of a gene is mutated, this is sufficient to cause the disease to be manifested.

Autosomal recessive inheritance pattern: The inheritance pattern whereby both copies of the gene are mutated and the person develops the condition because they have no normal copy. Carriers of recessive conditions are usually unaffected.

Autosomes: The chromosomes that are present in equal numbers in both male and female of the species (in humans, chromosomes 1 to 22).

Base pair: A pair of nucleotides, which are positioned opposite each other on the two strands of the DNA double helix. Adenine always pairs with thymine, and guanine with cytosine.

Carrier: A person who is generally not affected with the condition, but carries one faulty copy of a gene. Generally relates to heterozygotes in recessive or X-linked conditions.

CGH (comparative genomic hybridization): A molecular cytogenetic technique to ascertain gain and/or loss of base pairs in DNA. Sometimes called chromosomal CGH microarray analysis.

Chiasma: The point where two homologous chromosomes cross over during meiosis.

Chorionic villus biopsy: Removal of cells from the chorionic villi (developing placental tissue).

Chromatid: One of two lengths of chromosomal material (sister chromatids) that are joined at the centromere during cell replication. Each becomes a new chromosome.

Chromosome: The physical structures into which the DNA is packaged within the nucleus of cells. The usual number of chromosomes in humans is 46.

Clinical genetics: The branch of the health service that is chiefly involved in diagnosis of genetic conditions and genetic counseling for families.

Codon: A triplet in the messenger RNA that provides the code for one amino acid.

Colonoscopy: Investigation wherein the rectum, sigmoid and large colon are viewed directly via an endoscope.

Consanguinity: The biological relationship between two individuals who have a common ancestor.

Consultand: The person seeking genetic information, not necessarily the affected person in the family, who is usually called the proband.

Cordocentesis: Removal of a sample of fetal blood from the umbilical cord during pregnancy.

Cytogenetics: The study of chromosomes, in the laboratory.

Delay – developmental or learning delay: A term used to describe the failure of the child to reach milestones in physical, mental, emotional or social development within the expected age limits.

Deletion: The omission of a part of the genetic material; the term can be used in relation to either a gene or a chromosome.

Diploid: Having two copies of each autosome.

Disjunction: The separation of the replicated copies of the chromosomes into two daughter cells during the second stage of meiosis.

DNA: Deoxyribonucleic acid. The biochemical substance which forms the genome. It carries in coded form the information that directs the growth, development and function of physical and biochemical systems. It is usually present within the cell as two strands with a double helix formation (see *Chapter 4*).

Dominant: *See* Autosomal dominant.

Duplication: The abnormal repetition of a sequence of genetic material within a gene or chromosome.

Dysmorphic features: Physical features that are outside of the variability of the normal population. They may occur because of a change in the genetic code providing instructions for those features.

Eugenics: The study and practice of principles that will improve the genetic health and fitness of a population.

Exclusion test: A genetic test that uses samples from three generations of the family, to exclude the risk of a genetic disease or confirm a 50% or 25% risk.

Exon: A sequence of DNA that contributes to the protein product of a gene (*see also* Intron).

Expansion: An abnormally large repetition of specific DNA sequences within a gene.

Expression: The way in which the gene mutation is manifested within an individual.

FISH (fluorescent *in situ* hybridization): A technique that uses both cytogenetics and molecular biology to identify subtle changes in chromosome structure.

Gamete: Cell formed in the reproductive organs from the germline, in humans either ovum or sperm.

G-banding: A technique of staining the chromosomes to enable identification by creating a different pattern of bands along each chromosome.

Gene: The fundamental physical and functional unit of heredity consisting of a sequence of DNA.

Gene therapy: Therapy that is based upon the principle of replacing or modifying a faulty gene with a normal copy, in the relevant tissues. The aim is to reduce or obliterate the effects of the genetic condition.

Genetic counselor: A person whose main professional role is to offer information and support to clients who are concerned about a condition which may have a genetic basis.

Genetic screening: This term usually refers to population screening for a genetic variation or mutation.

Guthrie test: Blood test performed in the neonatal period to detect infants at high risk of phenylketonuria. A test for congenital hypothyroidism is usually performed at the same time.

Hemoglobinopathy: A genetic condition that affects the structure of the hemoglobin molecule.

Haploid: Having one copy of each autosome.

Heterogeneous: Pertaining to more than one gene.

Heterozygous: Having two different alleles at a genetic locus, usually one normal and one faulty copy of a gene (see also homozygous).

Homologous pair: Two copies of the same chromosome.

Homozygous: Having two identical alleles at a genetic locus. In Mendelian diseases these may be copies of a gene that are either both normal or both faulty.

Hybridization: Attachment of one DNA sequence to an identical sequence. Hybridization is used to attach a DNA probe to a segment of genomic DNA.

Hydrocephalus: The presence of excessive cerebrospinal fluid in the ventricles of the brain, normally leading to an enlarged head.

Imprinting: The phenomena whereby the two copies of a gene have a different function, depending upon their parental origin.

Induced abortion: Termination of pregnancy.

Insertion: The introduction of additional genetic material into a gene or chromosome.

Intron: A sequence of DNA that does not contribute to the code for protein product, as the genetic sequence within introns is omitted when the mRNA is made.

Inversion: An alteration in the sequence of genes along a particular chromosome. In a paracentric inversion, the change occurs on only one side of the centromere. In a pericentric inversion, the centromere is involved and material will move from the long to short arm and vice versa.

Karyotype: A description of the chromosome structure of an individual (assessed during metaphase), including the number of chromosomes and any variation from the normal pattern.

Linkage: The phenomenon whereby alleles that are physically close together on a chromosome will tend to be inherited together. This allows for a technique of genetic testing that tracks a specific copy of a gene through a family.

Locus: The position of a gene, a genetic marker or a DNA marker on a chromosome.

Maternal serum screening: A method of detecting a relative risk of Down syndrome in a pregnancy using biochemical testing of the mother's blood.

Meiosis: The production of gametes (haploid cells).

Mendelian disorder or **Mendelian condition:** A genetic disorder caused by a single gene fault, following a dominant, recessive or X-linked pattern of inheritance.

Messenger RNA: The sequence of base pairs that transfer the genetic code from the DNA to a functional protein.

Microdeletion: A minute deletion of chromosomal material that is usually not detectable using a microscope and has to be identified using a method such as FISH.

Mismatch repair gene: A gene whose function is to detect and repair errors in DNA transcription.

Mitochondrial DNA: The genetic material in the mitochondria, outside the nucleus of the cell.

Mitosis: The production of somatic diploid cells.

Molecular genetics: The study of genetic material at a molecular level, including DNA studies.

Monosomy: Having only one copy of a particular chromosome.

Mosaicism: Having more than one cell line with different chromosomes or expressing different genes.

Multifactorial: A condition is said to be multifactorial if both genetic and environmental influences are thought to be causative.

Mutation: A gene sequence variation that is found in less than 1% of the population. The mutation may cause a change in the protein product of the gene, and therefore cause health problems for the person concerned.

Neonatal death: The death of a baby who has shown signs of life, before the age of 28 days.

Neural tube defect: An abnormality of the spinal column or cranium (spina bifida or anencephaly).

New genetics: A term used to denote a change in the field of genetics, where the focus shifts from rare conditions caused by a fault in a single gene (including the 'Mendelian' conditions) to application of genetics to common diseases.

Non-directiveness: A model of counseling used in genetic counseling, which emphasizes the right of clients to make decisions without coercion from others.

Non-disjunction: Failure of the two copies of chromosomes to separate effectively into the two daughter cells.

PCR or **Polymerase chain reaction:** A laboratory method of manufacturing many copies of a sequence of DNA.

Pedigree: Family tree.

Penetrance: The extent to which specific gene mutations are manifested within an individual.

PGD or PIGD (preimplantation genetic diagnosis): A technique in which genetic testing of the embryos takes place after *in vitro* fertilization but prior to implantation. One or more unaffected embryos can then be introduced into the uterus.

Pharmacogenomics: The science of using the genetic variability in the population to target medication more effectively.

Polygenic: Relating to a number of different genes, e.g. a disorder is polygenic if it could be caused by a combination of mutations in several different genes.

Polymerase chain reaction: *See* PCR.

Polymorphism: Normal variation in sequence of DNA in a gene, differs from mutation in that it is usually found in more than 1% of the population.

Polyp: A small tumor growing from the surface of mucous membrane.

Population screening: Using a test to assess the risk or presence of a genetic disease in an entire section of the population, e.g. neonatal screening for hypothyroidism.

Proband: The affected person in the family or the person who is seeking genetic advice.

Probe: A sequence of manufactured DNA that attaches to an identical sequence in the genomic DNA for the purposes of genetic testing or research.

Recessive: *See* Autosomal recessive.

Reciprocal translocation: Exchange of chromosomal material between at least two chromosomes.

Recombination: The creation during meiosis of a new chromosome or sequence of DNA, which is a unique combination of the parent's maternal and paternal DNA.

Recurrence risk: The chance that a genetic condition will occur again in offspring or siblings of an affected person.

Restriction fragment length polymorphisms (RFLP): Fragments of DNA within a gene that have a normal variability in size when cut with specific enzymes.

Robertsonian translocation: An attachment of two acrocentric chromosomes end to end at the centromere.

Scanning: Investigation of physical structures using ultrasound device (sound waves).

Single nucleotide polymorphisms (SNPs): Polymorphic markers that detect single base changes in the DNA sequence.

Somatic: Relating to cells other than the germline.

Southern blotting: A laboratory method of DNA analysis.

Spina bifida: An interruption to the spinal column, with possible herniation of the spinal cord and meninges (myelomeningocoele). One form of neural tube defect (another being anencephaly).

Spontaneous abortion: Loss of a pregnancy without interference, miscarriage.

Stillbirth: A fetus of more than 24 weeks gestation who is born dead.

Syndrome: A number of physical features or abnormalities that fit a recognized pattern.

Teratogen: A substance that may harm the developing fetus.

Translocation: An alteration in the usual structure of a chromosome, wherein part or all of one chromosome is attached to another.

Trinucleotide repeat: A sequence of three bases that is repeated more than once at a site within a particular gene.

Trisomy: Having three copies of a particular chromosome.

Tumor suppressor gene: A gene whose normal function is to prevent the overgrowth or abnormal growth of cells.

Uniparental disomy: Inheritance of both copies of a particular chromosome from one parent only.

VNTR polymorphisms (variable number tandem repeats): Variations in the number of repeat sequences of DNA at a specific locus.

X-inactivation: In human females the early random inactivation of one of each of the X chromosomes, allowing expression of genes only on the active X chromosome.

X-linked inheritance pattern: A pattern of inheritance whereby the mutated gene is on the X chromosome, of which males have one copy and females have two.

References

1. Collins FS, McCusick VA (2001) Implications of the Human Genome Project for medical science. *JAMA* **285**: 540–544.
2. Pavlovic-Calic N, Muminhodzic K, Zildzic M, *et al.* (2007) Genetics, clinical manifestations and management of FAP and HNPCC. *Med Arh* **61**: 256–259.
3. Metcalfe KA, Birenbaum-Carmeli D, Lubinski J, *et al.* (2008) Hereditary Breast Cancer Clinical Study Group. International variation in rates of uptake of preventive options in BRCA1 and BRCA2 mutation carriers. *Int J Cancer* **122**: 2017–2022.
4. Shepherd M, Ellis I, Ahmad AM, *et al.* (2001) Predictive genetic testing in maturity-onset diabetes of the young (MODY). *Diabet Med* **18**: 417–421.
5. Wald NJ, Rodeck C, Hackshaw AK, Rudnicka A (2005) SURUSS in perspective. *Semin Perinatol* **29**: 225–235.
6. National Society of Genetic Counselors' Definition Task Force, Resta R, Biesecker BB, *et al.* (2006) A new definition of Genetic Counseling: National Society of Genetic Counselors' Task Force report. *J Genet Couns* **15**: 77–83.
7. Ad Hoc Committee on Genetic Counseling, American Society of Human Genetics (1975) Genetic counseling. *Am J Hum Genet* **27**: 240–242.
8. Eurogentest Project (2008) Recommendations For Genetic Counselling Related To Genetic Testing. Available at: www.eurogentest.org/professionals/info/public/unit3/final_recommendations_genetic_counselling.xhtml. [Accessed 3 January, 2009.]
9. Royal College of Physicians, Royal College of Pathologists and British Society for Human Genetics (2005) *Consent and Confidentiality in Genetic Practice: Guidance on Genetic Testing and Sharing Genetic Information*. Report of the Joint Committee on Medical Genetics. London: RCP, RCPath, BSHG.
10. United States Department of Health and Human Services. *Health Insurance Portability and Accountability Act (HIPPA)*. Available at: www.hhs.gov/ocr/hipaa/. [Accessed 28 October 2008.]
11. National Human Genome Research Institute. *Genetic Information Nondiscrimination Act*. Available at: www.genome.gov/10002077. [Accessed 28 October, 2008.]
12. Kessler S (1997) Psychological aspects of genetic counselling. XI. Nondirective-ness revisited. *Am J Med Genet* **72**: 164–171.
13. Kevles DJ (1985) *In the Name of Eugenics*. New York: Knopf/Pelican.
14. Shakespeare T (2006) Disability Rights. Available at: www.ukwatch.net/article/disability_rights. [Accessed 29 October, 2008.]
15. Rogers CR (1961) *On Becoming a Person*. London: Constable and Co Ltd.
16. Barker P (1998) *Basic Family Therapy*, 4th Edition. Oxford: Blackwell.
17. Jacobs M (1985) *The Presenting Past*. Milton Keynes: Open University Press.
18. Stewart I, Joines V (1987) *TA Today: A New Introduction to Transactional Analysis*. Nottingham: Lifespace Publishing.
19. AGNC Supervision Working Group (2007) Report from the UK and Eire Association of Genetic Nurses and Counsellors (AGNC) Supervision Working Group on Genetic Counselling Supervision. *J Gen Couns* **16**: 127–142.
20. Watson JD, Crick FH (1953) Molecular structure of nucleic acids: a structure for deoxyribonucleic acid. *Nature* **171**: 737–738.
21. Tijo H, Levan A (1956) The chromosomes of man. *Hereditas* **42**: 1–6.

22. Bejjani BA, Shaffer LG (2008) Clinical utility of contemporary molecular cytogenetics. *Annu Rev Genomics Hum Genet* **9**: 71–86.

23. Lander ES, Linton LM, Birren B, *et al.* (2001) Initial sequencing and analysis of the human genome. *Nature,* **409**: 860–921.

24. Venter JC, Adams MD, Myers EW, *et al.* (2001) The sequence of the human genome. *Science* **291**: 1304–1351.

25. Pearson TA, Manolio TA (2008) How to interpret a genome-wide association study. *JAMA* **299**: 1335–1344.

26. Gelb BD (2006) Marfan's syndrome and related disorders – more tightly connected than we thought. *N Engl J Med* **355**: 844–848.

27. Genome-based Research and Population Health Report of an expert workshop. Available at: www.graphint.org/ver2/. [Accessed 30 January 2009.]

28. Haddow J, Palomaki G (2004) ACCE: a model process for evaluating data on emerging genetic tests. In: Khoury M, Little J, Burke W (eds), *Human Genome Epidemiology*, pp. 217–233. Oxford: Oxford University Press.

29. Burke W, Zimmern R (2007) Moving beyond ACCE: An Expanded Framework for Genetic Test Evaluation. Available at: www.phgfoundation.org. [Accessed 12 January, 2009.]

30. United Kingdom Genetic Testing Network. Available at: www.ukgtn.nhs.uk/gtn/Home. [Accessed 12 January, 2009.]

31. Hogarth S, Javitt G, Melzer D (2008) The current landscape for direct-to-consumer genetic testing: legal, ethical, and policy issues. *Annu Rev Genomics Hum Genet* **9**: 161–182.

32. Patch C, Sequiros J, Cornel M (2009) Genetic horoscopes: is it all in the genes? Points for regulatory control of direct-to-consumer genetic testing. *Eur J Hum Genet,* advance online publication, 4 March 2009; doc: 10.1038/ejhg.2008.246.

33. MRC Vitamin Study Research Group (1991) Prevention of neural tube defects: results of the MRC vitamin study. *Lancet* **338**: 132–137.

34. De Wals P, Tairou F, Van Allen MI, *et al.* (2007) Reduction in Neural-Tube Defects after Folic Acid Fortification in Canada. *New Engl J Med* **357**: 135–142.

35. Eriksson UJ (1997) Embryo development in early pregnancy. In: Dornhurst A, Hadden D (eds), *Diabetes and Pregnancy.* Chichester: John Wiley and Sons.

36. Braude P, Flinter F (2007) Use and misuse of preimplantation genetic testing. *BMJ* **335**: 752–754.

37. PHGFoundation (2008) UK Human Fertilisation and Embryology Bill. Update available at: www.phgfoundation.org/news/4240/. [Accessed 1 January, 2009.]

38. Birsner ML, Farber JL, Berghella V (2008) Fatal aortic dissection in a patient with a family history of Marfan syndrome. *Obstet Gynecol* **112**: 472–475.

39. Lurie S, Manor M, Hagay ZJ (1998) The threat of type IV Ehlers-Danlos syndrome on maternal well-being during pregnancy: early delivery may make the difference. *J Obstet Gynaecol* **18**: 245–248.

40. Erez Y, Ezra Y, Rojansky N (2008) Ehlers-Danlos type IV in pregnancy. A case report and a literature review. *Fetal Diagn Ther* **23**: 7–9.

41. Georgy MS, Anwar K, Oates SE, Redford DH (1997) Perineal delivery in Ehlers-Danlos syndrome. *Br J Obstet Gynaecol* **104**: 505–506.

42. Koch R, Hanley W, Levy H, *et al.* (2000) Maternal phenylketonuria: an international study. *Mol Genet Metab* **71**: 233–239.

43. Sheard NF (2000) Importance of diet in maternal phenylketonuria. *Nutr Rev* **58**: 236–239.

44. Olson GL (1997) Cystic fibrosis in pregnancy. *Semin Perinatol* **21**: 307–312.

45. Tuck SM, Jensen CE, Wonke B, Yardumian A (1998) Pregnancy management and outcomes in women with thalassaemia major. *J Pediatr Endocrinol Metab* **11**: 923–928.

46. Aessopos A, Karabatsos F, Farmakis D, *et al.* (1999) Pregnancy in patients with well-treated beta-thalassaemia: outcomes for mothers and newborn infants. *Am J Obstet Gynecol* **180**: 360–365.

47. Daskalakis GJ, Papageorgiou IS, Antsaklis AJ, Michalas SK (1998) Pregnancy and homozygous beta thalassaemia major. *Br J Obstet Gynaecol* **105**: 1028–1032.

48. Balgir RS, Dash BP, Das RK (1997) Fetal outcome and childhood mortality in offspring of mothers with sickle cell trait and disease. *Indian J Pediatr* **64**: 79–84.

49. Mahomed K (2000) Prophylactic versus selective blood transfusion for sickle cell anaemia during pregnancy. *Cochrane Database Syst Rev* **2**: CD000040.

50. Arafeh JM, Baird SM (2006) Cardiac disease in pregnancy. *Crit Care Nurs Q* **29**: 32–52.

51. Gooding HC, Boehm K, Thompson RE, *et al.* (2002) Issues surrounding prenatal genetic testing for achondroplasia. *Prenat Diagn* **22**: 933–940.

52. Boue J, Boue A, Lazar P (1975) Retrospective and prospective epidemiological studies of 1500 karyotyped spontaneous human abortions. *Teratology* **12**: 11–26.

53. Brambati B (1990) Fate of human pregnancies. In: Edwards RG (ed.), *Establishing a Successful Human Pregnancy*, Serono Symposia **66**: 269–281. New York: Raven Press.

54. Council of Europe (1990) Committee of Ministers, Recommendation No. R (90) 13 on *Prenatal Genetic Screening, Prenatal Genetic Diagnosis and Associated Genetic Counselling* (June 21, 1990). Available at: www1.umn.edu/humanrts/instree/coerecr90-13.html. [Accessed 4 January, 2009.]

55. UK National Screening Committee (2003) *Antenatal screening – working standards incorporating those for the National Down Syndrome screening programme for England*. Available at: www.library.nhs.uk/screening/ViewResource.aspx?resID=33974&tabID=288&catID=1328. [Accessed 19 March, 2008.]

56. Skirton H, Barr O (2007) Influences on uptake of antenatal screening for Down syndrome: a review of the literature. *Evidence Based Midwifery* **5**: 4–9.

57. Public Health Foundation (2005) Available at: www.phgfoundation.org/news/2207/. [Accessed 19 March, 2008.]

58. Gilbert RE, Augood C, Gupta R, *et al.* (2001) Screening for Down's syndrome: effects, safety, and cost effectiveness of first and second trimester strategies. *BMJ* **323**: 423–425.

59. Wald NJ, Rodeck C, Hackshaw AK, Rudnicka A (2004) SURUSS in perspective. *Br J Obs Gynae* **111**: 521–531.

60. Chitty L, Kagan K, Molina F, *et al.* (2006) Fetal nuchal translucency scan and early prenatal diagnosis of chromosomal abnormalities by rapid aneuploidy screening: an observational study. *BMJ* **332**: 452–455.

61. Skirton H, Barr O (2008) Antenatal screening: informed consent and parental choice. Available at: www.learningdisabilities.org.uk/antenatal-screening/. [Accessed 4 January, 2009.]

62. Nanal R, Kyle P, Soothill PW (2003) A classification of pregnancy losses after invasive prenatal diagnostic procedures: an approach to allow comparison of units with a different case mix. *Prenat Diagn* **23**: 488–492.

63. Firth H (1991) Chorion villus sampling and limb deficiency – cause or coincidence? *Prenat Diag* **17**: 1313–1330.

64. Geifman-Holtzman O, Ober Berman J (2008) Prenatal diagnosis: update on invasive versus noninvasive fetal diagnostic testing from maternal blood. *Expert Rev Mol Diagn* **8**: 727–751.

65. Wright CF, Burton H (2008) The use of cell-free fetal nucleic acids in maternal blood for non-invasive prenatal diagnosis. *Hum Reprod Update* **15**: 139–151.

66. Ding C (2008) Maldi-TOF mass spectrometry for analyzing cell-free fetal DNA in maternal plasma. *Methods Mol Biol* **444**: 253–267.

67. Fan HC, Blumenfeld YJ, Chitkara U, *et al.* (2008) Noninvasive diagnosis of fetal aneuploidy by shotgun sequencing DNA from maternal blood. *Proc Natl Acad Sci USA* **105**: 16266–16271.

68. Draper ES, Rankin J, Tonks AM, *et al.* (2008) Recreational drug use: a major risk factor for gastroschisis? *Am J Epidemiol* **167**: 485–491.

69. Miyakoshi K, Ishimoto H, Tanigaki S, *et al.* (2001) Prenatal diagnosis of midgut volvulus by sonography and magnetic resonance imaging. *Am J Perinatol* **18**: 447–450.

70. Ryan AK, Goodship JA, Wilson DI, *et al.* (1997) Spectrum of clinical features associated with interstitial chromosome 22q11 deletions: a European collaborative study. *J Med Genet* **34**: 798–804.

71. Jacobs PA, Lelville M, Ratcliffe S, *et al.* (1974) A cytogenetic study of 11,680 newborn infants. *Ann Hum Genet* **37**: 359–376.

72. The President's Council on Bioethics (2008) *The Changing Moral Focus of Newborn Screening: An Ethical Analysis by the President's Council on Bioethics.* Available at: www.bioethics.gov/reports/newborn_screening/index.html. [Accessed 12 January, 2009.]

73. Skirton, H (2001) The client's perspective of genetic counseling – a grounded theory approach. *J Gen Couns* **10**: 311–330.

74. Clinical Genetics Society (1994) *The Genetic Testing of Children.* Available at: www.bshg.org.uk/documents/official_docs/testchil.htm. [Accessed 4 January, 2009.]

75. Hagerman PJ, Hagerman RJ (2004) The Fragile-X premutation: a maturing perspective. *Am J Hum Genet* **74**: 805–816.

76. Vercelli D (2008) Discovering susceptibility genes for asthma and allergy. *Nat Rev Immunol* **8**: 169–182.

77. Willer CJ, Speliotes EK, Loos RJ, *et al.* (2009) Six new loci associated with body mass index highlight a neuronal influence on body weight regulation. *Nat Genet* **41**: 25–34.

78. Cecil JE, Tavendale R, Watt P, *et al.* (2008) An obesity-associated FTO gene variant and increased energy intake in children. *N Engl J Med* **359**: 2558–2566.

79. Brady RO (2006) Enzyme replacement for lysosomal diseases. *Ann Rev Med* **57**: 283–296.

80. Knudson A (1971) Mutation and cancer: statistical study of retinoblastoma. *Proc Natl Acad Sci USA* **68**: 820–823.

81. Claus EB, Risch N, Thompson WD (1994) Autosomal dominant inheritance of early onset breast cancer. *Cancer* **73**: 643–651.

82. National Institute for Health and Clinical Excellence (NICE) *Familial Breast Cancer.* Available at: www.nice.org.uk/Guidance/CG41. [Accessed 8 December, 2008.]

83. Buys SS, Partridge E, Greene M, *et al.* (2005) Ovarian cancer screening in the prostate, lung, colorectal and ovarian (PLCO) cancer screening trial: findings from the initial screen of a randomized trial. *Am J Obstet Gynec* **193**: 1630–1639.

84. Bonis PA, Trikalinos TA, Chung M, *et al.* (2007) Hereditary nonpolyposis colorectal cancer: diagnostic strategies and their implications. *Evid Rep Technol Assess* **150**: 1–180.

85. Lovett E (1976) Family studies in cancer of the colon and rectum. *Br J Surg* **63**: 13–18.

86. Lynch J, Lynch HT (1994) Genetic counseling and HNPCC. *Anticancer Research* **14**: 1651–1656.

87. International Huntington Association. *Recommendations for Predictive Testing.* Available at: www.huntington-assoc.com/. [Accessed 3rd January, 2009.]

88. Skirton H, Glendinning N (1997) Using research to develop care for patients with Huntington's disease. *Br J Nurs* **6**: 83–90.

89. Harper PS (2004) *Practical Genetic Counselling,* 6th edition. London: Arnold.

90. Feder JN, Gnirke A, Thomas W, *et al.* (1996) A novel MHC class I-like gene is mutated in patients with hereditary haemochromatosis. *Nat Genet* **13**: 399–408.

91. Niederau C, Fischer R, Purschel A, *et al.* (1996) Long-term survival in patients with hereditary hemochromatosis. *Gastroenterology* **110**: 1107–1119.

92. Niederau C, Strohmeyer G, Stremmel W (1994) Epidemiology, clinical spectrum and prognosis of hemochromatosis. *Adv Exp Med Biol* **356**: 293–302.

93. Williams JK, Skirton H, Paulsen JS, Tripp-Reimer T (2009) The emotional experiences of family carers in Huntington disease. *J Adv Nurs* **65**: 789–798.

94. Mental Capacity Act (2005) Available at: www.opsi.gov.uk/ACTS/acts2005/ukpga_20050009_en_1. [Accessed 9 December, 2008.]

95. Yunis EJ, Zúñiga J, Koka PS, *et al.* (2006) Stem cells in aging: influence of ontogenic, genetic and environmental factors. *J Stem Cells* **1**: 125–147.

96. Yen K, Steinsaltz D, Mobbs CV (2008) Validated analysis of mortality rates demonstrates distinct genetic mechanisms that influence lifespan. *Exp Gerontol* **43**: 1044–1051.

97. Ostan R, Bucci L, Capri M, *et al.* (2008) Immunosenescence and immuno-genetics of human longevity. *Neuroimmunomodulation* **15**: 224–240.

98. Tonoki A, Kuranaga E, Tomioka T, *et al.* (2009) Genetic evidence linking age-dependent attenuation of the 26S proteasome with aging process. *Mol Cell Biol* **29**: 1095–1106.

99. Koropatnick TA, Kimbell J, Chen R, *et al.* (2008) A prospective study of high-density lipoprotein cholesterol, cholesteryl ester transfer protein gene variants, and healthy aging in very old Japanese-American men. *J Gerontol A Biol Sci Med Sci* **63**: 1235–1240.

100. Ross CA, Smith WW (2007) Gene–environment interactions in Parkinson's disease. *Parkinsonism Relat Disord* **13** (Suppl 3): S309–315.

101. Singh DK, Ahn B, Bohr VA (2008) Roles of RECQ helicases in recombination based DNA repair, genomic stability and aging. *Biogerontology* 2008 Dec 15 [Epub ahead of print].

102. Liu Y, Ordovas JM, Gao G, *et al.* (2009) Pharmacogenetic association of the APOA1/C3/A4/A5 gene cluster and lipid responses to fenofibrate: the genetics of lipid-lowering drugs and diet network study. *Pharmacogenet Genomics* **19**: 161–169.

103. Tan SH, Lee SC, Goh BC, Wong J (2008) Pharmacogenetics in breast cancer therapy. *Clin Cancer Res* **14**: 8027–8041.

104. Seeringer A, Kirchheiner J (2008) Pharmacogenetics-guided dose modifications of antidepressants. *Clin Lab Med* **28**: 619–626.

105. Gerretsen P, Pollock BG (2008) Pharmacogenetics and the serotonin transporter in late-life depression. *Expert Opin Drug Metab Toxicol* **4**: 1465–1478.

106. Skirton H, Frazier LQ, Calvin AO, Cohen MZ (2006) A legacy for the children – attitudes of older adults in the United Kingdom to genetic testing. *J Clin Nurs* **15**: 565–573.

107. Frazier L, Calvin AO, Mudd GT, Cohen MZ (2006) Understanding of genetics among older adults. *J Nurs Scholarsh* **38**: 126–132.

108. Darwin C (1859) *The Origin of Species*. London: Dent edition, published 1972.

109. Galton F (1874) *English Men of Science, their nature and nurture*. London: Macmillan.

110. Galton F (1892) *Hereditary Genius*, 2nd Edition. London: Macmillan.

111. Galton F (1897) *The Average Contribution of Each Several Ancestor to the Total Heritage of the Offspring*. London: Royal Society Proceedings.

112. Blacker C (c. 1945) *Eugenics in Retrospect and Prospect*. Glasgow: The University Press.

113. Garrod AE (1909) *Inborn Errors of Metabolism*. London: Oxford Medical Publications, Hodder and Stoughton.

114. Carter CO, Fraser Roberts JA, Evans KA, Buck AR (1971) Genetic clinic: a follow-up. *Lancet* **1**: 281–285.

115. Skirton H, Barnes C, Curtis G, Walford-Moore J (1997) The role and practice of the genetic nurse: report of the AGNC Working Party. *J Med Genet* **34**: 141–147.

116. Plasschaert A, Boyd M, Andrieu S (2002) Development of professional competences. *Eur J Dent Educ.* **6** (Suppl. 3): 33–44. Available at: www.blackwell-synergy.com/doi/pdf/10.1034/j.1600-0579.6.s3.5.x?cookieSet=1. [Accessed 4 January, 2009.]

117. Eurogentest Project (2008) Core competences in genetics for health professionals in Europe. Available at: www.eurogentest.org/professionals/documents/info/public/unit6/core_competences.xhtml. [Accessed 3 January, 2009.]

118. Greco K, Prows CA, Skirton H, *et al.* (2006) *Genetics/Genomics Nursing: Scope and Standards of Practice.* International Society of Nurses in Genetics and American Nurses Association.

119. Genetic Counsellor Registration Board (2006) *Registration.* Available at: www.agnc.org.uk/Registration/registration.htm. [Accessed 3 January, 2009.]

Answers to 'Test yourself' questions

Chapter 1

A1. The five main components of a genetic counseling interaction are:

i)   taking and recording the family medical history (including drawing the family tree) and confirming relevant diagnoses

ii)   making an assessment of the risk of developing the condition for an individual or for future family members

iii)   providing information about the condition, the mode of inheritance and current methods of management or prevention

iv)   discussing the options available to the individual in the context of his or her own personal circumstances

v)   providing psychosocial support to facilitate the individual to make informed choices and to adapt to the risk or the condition

A2. The difference between a diagnostic and pre-symptomatic test is that a diagnostic test is offered when the individual already has signs or symptoms of the condition. The test is therefore often performed to confirm what is already suspected by the healthcare team, as well as by the individual and/ or the family. A diagnostic genetic test may not differ in any substantive way from other diagnostic tests, for example, by diagnosing polycystic kidney disease using ultrasound to detect cysts in the kidney, whereas a pre-symptomatic test is performed for an individual who is at genetic risk of the condition but is not yet showing signs or symptoms. A pre-symptomatic test therefore gives an indication of the person's genetic status, confirming whether or not they have inherited the gene mutation and will or will not go on to develop the disease.

The client's reaction to a positive result may well vary, depending on whether the test was diagnostic or pre-symptomatic. Because a pre-symptomatic test conveys information about the individual's future, it may have long-lasting implications for the way he or she lives, for example, by allowing planning with respect to career and having a family. Because of protocols, those having a pre-symptomatic test have usually had to think carefully about the decision to be tested. While many psychologically prepare themselves 'for the worst', they may be less prepared for a result that eliminates the chance of them developing the condition and respond with disbelief or guilt. However, not everyone who has a diagnostic test is aware of symptoms and a diagnostic test result can sometimes be more surprising to the individual than a pre-symptomatic test result would be.

A3. Based on the referral letter for the Spencer family, the family might be experiencing the following types of loss prior to a genetic appointment:
i)   loss of the ability to communicate easily with Luke
ii) loss of some of their aspirations for Luke's future
iii) loss of confidence in their own reproductive abilities
iv) loss of confidence in having another child

Chapter 2

A1. Practice drawing a family tree by doing your own.

A2. The chance that Martin is a carrier of the condition is 1 in 3; his mother has a 2 in 3 chance of being a carrier and he has half her risk.

At birth, Martin's mother would have been considered to have a 1 in 4 chance of inheriting two copies of the mutation (one from each parent), in which case she would have been affected. She had a 1 in 4 chance of having no copy of the mutation and 2 chances out of 4 of being a carrier. However, as we now know that she is not affected, her carrier risk alters to 2 chances out of 3.

A3. Bernice's father was born with a 1 in 2 or 50% chance of inheriting the condition. However, if he is now in his 50s and has no sign of the condition, his chance of having the mutation is less than 50%. Because hypertrophic cardiomyopathy could still affect him at an older age, it is hard to quantify that risk, but Bernice's risk is less than 25%.

The knowledge that Bernice's father died in a traffic accident at the age of 29 years, does not affect Bernice's risk because we have no information about the state of Bernice's father's heart when he died.

A4. The following points should be considered in your reflection:
- family trees are sensitive confidential information
- each individual in a family may hold different information at different levels of knowledge
- families may not have accurate information about a diagnosis in other members

Chapter 4

A1. The oocytes that form the eggs are present in the ovary from before birth. It is thought that the process of meiosis becomes less efficient as the cells age. It is therefore more likely that an unbalanced number of chromosomes will be present in the egg of a woman over 40 years of age, compared to a younger woman.

A2. The change to the normal human chromosome pattern designated by the following:

a) 47,XXY is Klinefelter syndrome. The male inherits an additional copy of the X chromosome.

b) 47,XY,+13 is Trisomy 13 or Patau syndrome. The fertilized egg contains an additional copy of chromosome 13.

c) 47,XY,+21 is Trisomy 21 or Down syndrome. The fertilized egg contains an additional copy of chromosome 21.

d) 45,XX,der(13;14)(p11;q11) is the Robertsonian translocation of chromosomes 13 and 14.

e) As one copy of chromosome 13 is attached to one copy of chromosome 14, the total number of chromosomes counted is 45 rather than 46.

A3. Using ISCN nomenclature, the following would be described in a cytogenetic report as:

a) 46,XX which is a normal female chromosome arrangement

b) 47,XX,+18 or 47,XY,+18 which are chromosome arrangements indicative of Edwards syndrome

c) 45,X which is a chromosome arrangement indicative of Turner syndrome

A4.

a) For a neonate suspected of having a sub-microscopic microdeletion of chromosome 22q11, a routine karyotype would be carried out but this is unlikely to show the microdeletion, as the deletion is too small to be detected using a microscope. Analysis of the relevant portion of the long arm of chromosome 22 using a FISH probe will usually enable the microdeletion to be identified. CGH arrays may be used routinely in the future for checking for small imbalances in chromosomal material.

b) To provide the parents with details of the risk of recurrence, the following advice could be given:

■ The microdeletion could have occurred sporadically, in the egg or sperm that contributed to that particular child. If that is the case, the risk of a future child inheriting the condition is low.

■ However, the child may have inherited the microdeletion from one of the parents. For this reason, the parents should have a karyotype and FISH analysis of their chromosomes. Even if the parents have no signs of the condition this should be done, as the condition has variable expression and the signs may be very subtle.

■ If one of the parents has the microdeletion, the chance of any future child inheriting it is 50%. Parents who have normal chromosomes will be informed that they still have some recurrence risk (usually several per cent) because of the chance of germinal mosaicism, which occurs when a number of germ cells in either the ovary or testis have the microdeletion.

A5. The PCR process involves replicating a segment of DNA many times. A substantial number of copies from the original sample can be produced for testing and so only a small initial sample is required.

Chapter 5

A1. The following criteria can be used to evaluate a genetic test before it is offered within a healthcare setting:
- analytical validity – does it measure what it says it measures
- clinical validity – is it linked to the disorder that you are interested in and how does the test perform in a clinical population
- clinical utility – what is its usefulness
- ethical legal and social aspects

Chapter 6

A1. Issues to discuss with a couple with mild learning disability planning on having a baby, would include the following:
- components of a healthy diet
- lifestyle issues that may affect the fetus and mother, such as smoking, or use of alcohol or other substances
- medications prescribed for or being taken by the mother (such as anti-convulsant therapy)
- the recommendation for the woman to take folic acid supplements pre-conceptually and for the first 3 months of pregnancy
- the possibility of screening for congenital abnormalities or other conditions in the fetus (such as Rhesus disease) during pregnancy.

A2. The recommendations for pre-conceptual folic acid supplementation are:
- for a woman with no history of neural tube defect, usually in the order of 0.04 – 0.05 mg per day
- for a woman who has had a child with spina bifida, usually in the order of 0.4 – 0.5mg per day

Chapter 7

A1. When present at the delivery of a baby with abnormalities, to avoid creating fear in the parents, nurses and midwives may discuss the baby's features realistically as follows.
- It may be helpful to begin with those features that are normal, describing the baby's arms and legs, for example, and saying that the baby has the usual number of fingers and toes. Showing the parents the normal features may give them some reassurance, as they may dread seeing what they believe is a grossly abnormal child.
- For those features that are unusual, using concrete terms could be helpful to the parents. For example, 'the eyes are blue but the shape is

different to usual, they slant slightly upwards' or 'the baby's neck is shorter than usual'.

A2. For consent to be informed, the woman must understand the information provided, have capacity to make a judgement and be able to communicate her decision. The professional cannot force her to listen to an explanation, but has a duty of care to ensure that she is giving informed consent before administering the test. It may be helpful to ask her to explain what she understands about what the test involves, limitations of the test and implications of the result. The midwife then needs to make a judgement about whether the conditions for consent have been met.

A3. When the parents of a stillborn baby do not consent to a post-mortem, information can still be recorded by:

- carefully examining the baby and recording all normal and abnormal features
- taking photographs of the baby's features (with parental consent) for the medical record
- suggesting, if possible, that a geneticist or experienced pediatrician is asked to examine the baby (with parental consent)

Chapter 8

A1. A newborn with a sub-mucous cleft could have a 22q11 microdeletion, so you would ask if other members of the family had a history of:

- cleft palate
- learning difficulties (including speech delay)
- congenital heart defect
- metabolic disturbances in the neonatal period (babies with 22q11 may have hypocalcemia)
- immune disorders (possibly due to thymic hypoplasia and/or T cell deficiency)

Of course, the sub-mucous cleft could be sporadic or due to another genetic condition, so the parents should also be asked whether there is a family history of other congenital abnormalities.

A2. The lack of family history can be explained to parents as follows. Every individual carries some gene faults, but as we have two copies of most of our genes, if that person also has a normal copy of the gene, they will not experience health problems connected with the faulty gene. Each parent donates one copy of each gene to their child. If the child inherits a faulty copy from the mother and a faulty copy from the father, he or she will have no normal copy and will develop the condition. Most people are unaware they are carriers and members of both sides of the family could have been carriers of the faulty gene for many generations without ever having an affected child.

A3. A malformation occurs when a tissue or organ develops abnormally because of a genetic or environmental influence (or both). Examples of malformations include: congenital heart defect due to 22q11 microdeletion, cleft lip or palate due to a single gene disorder, skeletal abnormalities due to achondroplasia, but there are of course many others.

Deformation occurs when a tissue or organ begins to develop normally, but the development is altered by some external influence (such as a teratogen or maternal infection). Examples of deformation include: talipes, immature pulmonary development due to oligohydramnios, or deafness due to rubella infection during pregnancy.

Chapter 9

A1. Joe is an adult and has the right to make his own decision – Marie has no rights to force him to give a sample. Informed consent should be sought from Joe if possible and it should be assumed he has the ability to consent unless it is shown otherwise.

Joe should not be coerced into giving a sample, however, it should be explained to him that he may help Marie by giving a sample. He has the same rights as anyone else to decide to act altruistically for the benefit of his sister.

The unborn children have no rights in this situation.

If Joe was 10 years old his parents may be able to consent on his behalf if they felt it was in his best interests. Assent from Joe to have the sample taken should still be sought.

A2. The accepted terms for the following features are:
a) hypertelorism – widely spaced eyes
b) short philtrum – shorter than usual distance between the nose and upper lip
c) right sided polydactyly – additional finger on the right hand
d) bilateral 2/3 syndactyly – webbing between the 2nd and 3rd fingers on both hands

A3. The following terms mean:
a) hypotelorism – the space between the eyes is narrower than usual
b) brachydactyly – fingers and/or toes shorter than usual
c) macroglossia – large tongue
d) epicanthic folds – additional folds of skin on the inner canthus of the eye

Chapter 10

A1. There is generally no legal duty of care to someone who is not your patient but professionals may feel they have an ethical duty to try to inform the relatives of their risk. However, if the proband does not wish their relatives to be informed, the professionals are unable to do this as they would be breaking the confidentiality of the original patient. Discussion over time with the proband may facilitate her to disclose the information to her sisters.

A2. In general it is not usual to test the son or daughter of a person affected with an autosomal recessive condition, because the risk to the offspring is very low. However, the risk would be higher if there is a history of the condition on both sides of the family, or if the affected man had been married to a biological relative. In the case of hemachromatosis, a genetic test would not necessarily indicate if the person was actually affected, whereas taking a measurement of the blood iron levels would indicate if treatment was required.

A3. It is important to consider whether the couple might be influenced by their experience of the condition in the family (for example, whether or not the treatment was successful in affected relatives), pressure from within the family to have prenatal testing, their own attitudes to the condition, and their attitudes to termination of pregnancy.

Chapter 11

A1. There are many discoveries that have informed our understanding of the influence of genes on the aging process, including:
- the genes that influence the inflammatory processes (inflammaging)
- apoptosis (controlled cell death)
- the function of proteosome 26S, which has an impact on the rate of neurodegeneration

A2. The group of genes known to be involved in the metabolism of drugs used in the treatment of depression are the cytochrome group. Two specific genes of major influence are CYP2D6 and CYP2C19.

A3. A test for variants of the gene influencing lipoprotein metabolism may provide valuable information on the most effective method of treating the patient to reduce his or her triglyceride levels.

Appendix 1

1. Jason's chance is 5/105 or less than 5%.

2. Mike's chance is 30/130 or 23%.

Appendix 2

1. The partner with no family history will have a chance of 1/120 of being a carrier. Any future child of the couple will have a $1/120 \times 1 \times 1/4 = 1/480$ chance of inheriting the condition.

Appendix 1

The Bayesian calculation

The Bayesian calculation is based on both the prior information (risk based on the family history) and conditional probability relating to information obtained by testing or based on other factors such as the person's current age. A likelihood ratio is obtained which can easily be converted to a risk estimate.

Step 1

What is the prior probability?

(a) Risk of being affected/a carrier

(b) Risk of not being affected/a carrier

Step 2

What is the conditional probability (based on additional information)?

(A) Chance of this result if affected/a carrier

(B) Chance of this result if not affected/a carrier

Step 3

Determine the joint probability.

Multiply a $\times$ A

Multiply b $\times$ B

Express a $\times$ A as a ratio of b $\times$ B

Step 4

Convert ratio to final probability expressed as a fraction or percentage.

It is easiest to demonstrate using an example.

Case 1

In a clinical example, William has adult polycystic kidney disease (APKD). He asks about the risk of his son Harry (aged 30 years) having APKD. This is an autosomal dominant condition so Harry's prior risk is 1/2. However, he has a kidney scan which shows no cysts. Only 2% of those inheriting the faulty gene for APKD will have no cysts at the age of 30 years, so this information can be used to modify Harry's risk.

Step 1

(a) Prior risk of Harry having APKD = 1/2

(b) Prior risk of Harry not having APKD = 1/2

Step 2

(A) Risk of negative scan result if Harry has APKD = 2% = 1/50 (because 98% of those affected would have cysts, this is the chance of a false negative result)

(B) Risk of negative scan result if Harry has inherited APKD = 1 (because all those non-affected will have a negative result)

Step 3

Calculate likelihood of Harry having APKD and of him not having APKD

Likelihood of having APKD	Likelihood of not having APKD
$1/2 \times 1/50 = 1/100$	$1/2 \times 1 = 1/2$
$= 1/100$	$= 50/100$

Likelihood ratio of 1: 50 that Harry has APKD

Remember that this is a ratio and not a fraction; add both numbers together to obtain the denominator for the fraction.

Harry's chance of having APKD is 1/51 (less than 2%)

Case 2

Colin is born with a 2/3 chance of being a carrier of cystic fibrosis. He has a genetic carrier test that detects 90% of mutations found in carriers of cystic fibrosis in our population.

	Carrier	Not a carrier
Prior probability	2/3	1/3
Conditional probability	1/10	1
Joint probability	2/30 = 1/15	1/3 = 5/15
Final probability	1/6	5/6

The chance that Colin is a carrier is 1/6 or about 17%.

Case 3

Ruth has a 25% chance of being a carrier of DMD. However, she has a serum creatine kinase test that indicates her chance of being a carrier is raised. Only 15% of non-carriers would have a CK result in the same range.

	Carrier	Not carrier
Prior probability	1/4	3/4
Conditional probability	85/100	15/100
Joint probability	85/400	45/400
Final probability	85/130	45/130

The additional information has tilted the balance in favour of Ruth being a carrier of DMD. Ruth's has a 65% chance of being a carrier.

As it is usually only boys who are significantly affected with DMD, and as she has two possible X chromosomes to hand on, there is a 1 in 4 risk of the fetus having the condition, in each pregnancy. The risk that Ruth will have an affected boy in her next pregnancy is $65/100 \times 1/4 = 65/400$. This translates into a percentage risk of 16%.

Here are some problems for you to try.

Q1. Jason is born with a 50% chance of having inherited retinitis pigmentosa (X-linked form). He has annual eye examinations, including an electroretinograph (ERG). In this type of X-linked RP, over 95% of those affected who have inherited the gene mutation will have changes detected in the retina by the age of 25 years. Jason is 28 years old and has no such changes. What is Jason's chance of having inherited retinitis pigmentosa?

Q2. Mike's father died of bowel cancer at 27 years of age. His father's father also had bowel cancer diagnosed at the age of 35 years. Mike has been told that he has a 50% chance of having inherited a gene mutation that would predispose him to bowel cancer. His blood sample is tested for mutations known to be associated with hereditary non-polyposis colon cancer (HNPCC), but no mutation is found. The tests that have been done are thought to detect a total of 70% of mutation carriers. What is the chance that he has inherited a mutation from his father?

Appendix 2

Using the Hardy–Weinberg equilibrium

The Hardy–Weinberg equilibrium states that $p^2 + 2pq + q^2 = 1$, where p is the gene frequency of the normal allele and q is the gene frequency of the mutated allele of a particular gene. If q is the gene frequency of a mutated recessive gene, then the frequency of carriers of the recessive gene is $2pq$. In reality, because the population sample is so large, the frequency of the normal allele (p) is regarded as 1. Therefore for practical purposes the carrier rate in the population (frequency of **heterozygotes**) is $2q$.

Usually the frequency of **homozygotes** (number of affected people) in a population is known, and this figure can be used to calculate carrier frequency.

Take, for example, a population where 1 in 1600 children is born with cystic fibrosis.

The number of homozygotes with the recessive condition (q^2) is 1 in 1600

$q = 1/40$ (the square root of $1/1600$)
$2q = 1/20$

The carrier risk for someone with no family history of cystic fibrosis in this population is therefore 1 in 20.

This information can be used to assess the risk of a couple having a baby with a recessive condition. The risk is calculated by multiplying

the carrier risk of the father
by
the carrier risk of the mother
by
the chance of the child inheriting the faulty copy of the gene from both parents (1 in 4).

Try the following example.

Q1. In a particular population the number of children born with spinal muscular atrophy (SMA) is 1 per 14 400 children. What is the chance that a person with no known family history of SMA will carry the condition? What is the risk of having a child with SMA for a couple where one partner is known to be a carrier and the other has no family history of SMA?

Appendix 3

Southern blotting

Southern blotting (named after its inventor Ed Southern) was the first method of analysis of DNA that utilized hybridization. The technique can be used on large fragments of DNA, which are too large to be amplified in a PCR reaction.

The DNA is cut into fragments using restriction enzymes that will only cut at specific sequences of bases, e.g. after a CTG sequence. The DNA is extracted from the cell and cut into fragments; because the restriction enzyme cuts at specific sites, a number of different-sized fragments are produced and these are called **restriction fragment length polymorphisms (RFLPs)**. The length of these RFLPs may be altered by a mutation. The fragments are separated by size using gel electrophoresis (*Figure*). Because the fragments are slightly negatively charged they move from the negative end of the gel to the positive end, with the larger fragments moving more slowly than the smaller fragments. The fragments are then denatured in alkali to make them single-stranded and are then transferred to a nitrocellulose membrane by blotting. A labeled DNA probe is hybridized to the membrane. If the probe is radioactively labeled, the membrane is analyzed by autoradiography, with the result being a film which reveals a number of bands corresponding to the fragments to which the probe has hybridized. A specific mutation can be detected if it alters a restriction enzyme cutting site, so that the presence of a mutation causes a different band pattern to that observed in the absence of a mutation. Large deletions or insertions will also change the length of the restriction fragments.

Southern blotting has also been used extensively in research to isolate genes and track them through families. Southern blotting analyzes DNA, whereas another similar technique, Northern blotting, is used to analyze RNA.

Genomic DNA is obtained from a sample of tissue (usually blood)

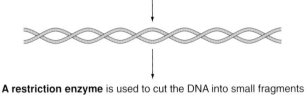

A restriction enzyme is used to cut the DNA into small fragments

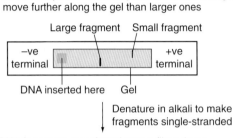

The fragments are subjected to electrophoresis. Smaller fragments move further along the gel than larger ones

Large fragment   Small fragment

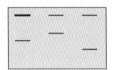

−ve terminal   +ve terminal

DNA inserted here   Gel

Denature in alkali to make fragments single-stranded

DNA fragments transferred onto a filter sheet.
Filter sheet is put into a bath of radioactive probes

After the probes have attached to specific DNA fragments, the filter sheet is analyzed by an autoradiography

Figure. Technique used in Southern blotting.

Index